ARE YOU POISONING YOUR PETS?

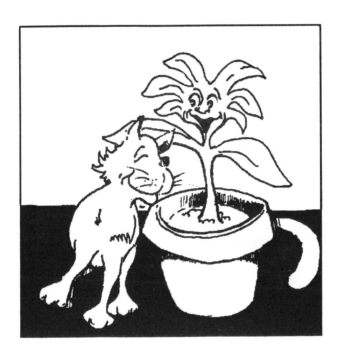

A GUIDEBOOK TO PET HEALTH AND SANITY

NINA ANDERSON AND HOWARD PEIPER
ILLUSTRATED BY RICHARD VAIL

Published by SAFE GOODS
East Canaan, Connecticut

ARE YOU POISONING YOUR PETS? is not intended as medical advice. It is written solely for informational and educational purposes. Please consult a health professional should the need for one be indicated.

ARE YOU POISONING YOUR PETS?

ISBN 1-884820-14-X
Library of Congress Catalog Card Number: 95-068436

Printed in the United States of America

Edited by William Reeves

Published by Safe Goods
283 East Canaan Rd. (PO Box 36)
East Canaan, CT 06024

PREFACE

I believe you are about to read a very informative, well written book about a subject which unfortunately, gets little thought or attention. The common place, every day products and substances which are purchased for ourselves, our homes and for our companion animals, often-times have hidden dangers. To be even more direct, some of these products are dangerous and even life threatening!

High powered advertising agencies have the incredible knack of driving consumers to purchase these products without ever mentioning their potential toxic properties. The authors have compiled an eye-opening, well written, comprehensive summary of potentially toxic substances. The book begins with information on dangerous pesticides and cleaning products and continues with serious poisons, such as anti-freeze and carbon monoxide. It finishes on an up-beat note, with a discussion of diet, life giving foods, supplements and remedies for your animal companion.

In a time when chronic disease conditions of animals, such as Cancer, Arthritis, Diabetes, AIDS, etc., are on the up-swing and nearly in an "epidemic" state, this book opens the door to some possible underlying causes. Perhaps, we should spend more time eliminating these materials from our home and environment and take special note of what happens... to the incidence of chronic degenerative diseases such as cancer, in both people and animals.

-Robert S. Goldstein, VMD

(Dr. Goldstein is a holistic veterinarian, practicing in New York State, and is co-editor, with his wife, Susan, of "Health Animals", a holistic companion animal newsletter published by Phillips Publishing of Potomac, MD.)

INTRODUCTION

There is ever increasing public awareness regarding the effect our lifestyles have on our pet's health. Are we poisoning them with chemical cleaners, pesticides, air fresheners and building or decorating materials? In recent times, the media has looked for answers about human health issues, and uncovered volumes of information on the subject of indoor air pollution. This research was not made available to the public, most likely to avoid confrontation with manufacturers of synthetic building and decorating materials.

For instance, a Journal of the American Medical Association reports a forty five percent higher incidence of respiratory infection among occupants of new buildings than those of older ones. They have not done studies concerning the effects on the millions of pets living in these buildings. The primary suspect comes from recent energy-efficient construction methods which make houses so well insulated that no air leaks in or out. While this saves lots of dollars in heating costs, it also traps chemical fumes within the home. Since this is where your pet spends a good bit of time, they may be developing health problems because of this polluted air.

Dangerous fumes come from many of the newer building materials which use a variety of toxic adhesives, plastics, fire retardant sprays, and paint containing volatile organic chemicals. Also captured within this "tight house" are mold spores which lurk in damp areas, heating systems, humidifiers, carpets and dust. Carbon monoxide from faulty heating systems also has a greater chance of existing in lethal dosages within poorly ventilated structures.

Veterinarians are seeing more cases of cancer in animals as well as behavioral problems and poisonings. It could be that something is happening within our closed well-insulated houses that we haven't looked at yet. If we are building or decorating with new materials containing formaldehyde, plastics, synthetics, petroleum products, etc., all leaching these fumes into the indoor air, then we should put gas masks on our pets. Cats especially have difficulty eliminating toxic chemicals, because their systems are inefficient at metabolizing foreign intruders.

Older homes have their own risks to health, primarily because before 1978 paint contained lead. This can cause problems, especially in puppies who may either chew painted wood or breathe lead dust. Household cleaners can be extremely toxic to pets as well as our common bug sprays and garden pesticides.

Many books have been written about healthy houses and their associated health implications to humans. The television media has covered stories about toxic carpets and lead paint ingestion. Everyday, newspapers or magazines report on the tragedies of carbon monoxide poisoning in the home. Health articles concerned with mold allergies are prolific during the start of the heating season.

People are aware that these problems exist, but few realize how hazardous your consumer lifestyle is to your pets. This book was written on the assumption that you will treat it as a guide to prevent pet sickness, by being responsible in your use of toxic household products. With proper testing, identification and verification you can eliminate many of these hazards. And...if you want to reduce the effects of the contaminant, we have provided some economical solutions.

Should extensive remediation be necessary to fix a problem, then it is advisable to contact a professional company that specializes in the area you wish to treat. Every home can have the newest of luxuries and healthy pets if the proper precautions are taken. If you are remodeling or redecorating, we advise you to explore alternatives to chemical based products.

TABLE OF CONTENTS

PESTICIDES AND FLEAS

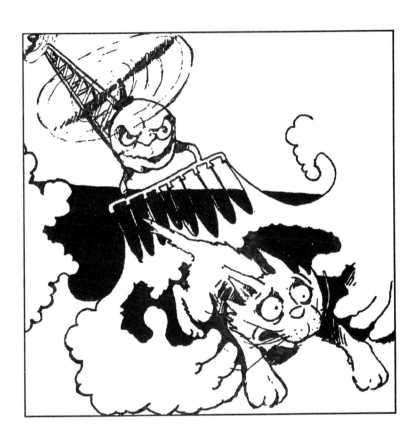

Our lifestyles tend to make many of us hate bugs and dirt. Therefore we will do most anything to rid our homes and yards of these creatures, whether they are beneficial or not. Unfortunately we do not realize the toll to our health and our pets' health from all these toxic substances.

Pesticides used to control weeds, insects especially fleas and ticks, termites, rodents and fungi, are sold as sprays, liquids, sticks, powder, crystals, balls and foggers. There are more than 34,000 pesticides in use and they are the number two cause in the U.S. of household poisonings in humans. People don't intentionally ingest pesticides, therefore statistics may be more alarming for dogs and cats who indiscriminately eat toxic-laden substances and groom them from their fur.

Insecticides as well as plastics' ingredients and particulate from household detergents can disrupt an animal's biological processes. This can manifest itself by feminizing male animals, and disrupting their ability to reproduce. In a Florida study from 1985-1990, 67 per cent of male panthers were born with one or more undescended testes, fostering infertility. They found these animals had twice as much estrogen as testosterone. Cause was assumed to come from "estrogenic" chemicals, primarily pesticides. Female seagulls were found to be sharing nests with other females and were not interested in mating. These situations are critical in the wild as it further decimates endangered species.

Although our cats and dogs are not in danger of extinction, long-term exposure to these toxins may cause chronic disease, therefore we must be more responsible in our treatment of bugs and dirt.

SYMPTOMS OF
PESTICIDE POISONING

BIRDS

LISTLESSNESS
SIDE TO SIDE HEAD MOVEMENTS
HEAD TREMORS
ERRATIC FLIGHT
PARALYSIS
RESPIRATORY FAILURE
RUFFLED FEATHERS
DROOPING WINGS
REGURGITATION

DOGS & CATS

INFERTILITY
SEXUAL ORGAN DEFORMITY
IRRITABILITY
CANCER
FOAMING OF MOUTH
INCREASED RESPIRATORY RATE
SEIZURES
STIFFNESS
CONVULSIONS
GASTROENTERITIS
DEPRESSION
COLIC
ANOREXIA
WEAKNESS
NAUSEA/VOMITING
NERVOUSNESS
WATERY DIARRHEA

3

LAWN CHEMICALS

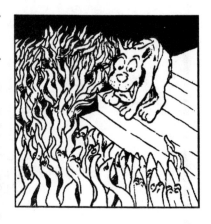

Approximately 91 percent of all American households apply 300 million pounds of pesticides annually. Most are insoluble in water and therefore stay around a long time and can poison your cat or dog. The most potent and widely used weed killer is 2,4,D and has been proven to have effects on humans such as depression, loss of memory, paranoia, irritability and cancer. Again, verification of many of these symptoms came from animal studies, therefore our poor pets can exhibit the same symptoms.

Lawn fertilizers, weed and insect killers can contain chloropyrifos, diazinon, 2,4,D, banvel, benomyl and daconil, all considered hazardous to human health. A study reported in the Journal of the National Cancer Institute found that dogs exposed to repeated applications of 2,4,D herbicide were twice as likely to get malignant lymphoma. Toxic weed killers should never be used by pet owners whose animals go outside and come in contact with the areas contaminated. Investigate natural pest control methods which may have a less toxic effect on your pet, or dig the weeds out by hand.

AGRICULTURAL AND TREE SPRAYING

Agricultural spraying can affect any animal caught in the line of fire. If they drink water into which the pesticides have leached they may be affected, although it is more difficult to determine the cause. DDT, Chlordane and Lindane are some common names for these potential illers. They remain in the air and on the ground for years.

For example, Chlordane has a half-life of 50 years and was banned from termite pesticides by the EPA in 1980. DDE, a by-product of DDT, is assumed to have been ingested through contaminated food by some women with breast cancer, whose tumors contained the pesticide. Female animals can be at risk as well. Not only can they eat food sprayed with pesticides, but may ingest it by breathing air from recently sprayed areas, and grooming their fur.

Contaminated animals can exhibit foaming of the mouth, irritability, increased respiratory rate and even seizures. If proper treatment is not administered immediately the animal can die. Dogs are more susceptible to airborne contamination through breathing, whereas cats readily ingest toxins because they lick the fur on which the toxin has landed.

GARDEN CHEMICAL SPRAYS

We may feel successful if we grow a good crop of vegetables or a beautiful flower garden all free from insects, but do we consider the hazard to birds and animals from our use of pest control insecticides?

Our wild birds are at our mercy. We kindly feed them all winter, just to make them sick in the summer by spraying our fruits and vegetables. Airborne contaminants can infect birds and even more toxic are the flower nectars and seeds used as food. Laced with the residue from pesticides, birds are eating poisonous meals. It is very important to feed wild birds a seed without additives or fillers and to continue feeding them healthy seed, year round.

Cats and dogs are not immune to insect sprays. Not only can they be affected through ingestion of contaminated food, but from direct contact with the pesticide as well. Any animal rummaging around in the garden, whether it be your dog or a stray rabbit or raccoon may become covered in spray residue. This can give them a skin disorder and can affect their internal organs when they groom their fur.

SYMPTOMS FROM PESTICIDES

The chemicals in pesticides are fat soluble and are stored in the fatty tissues, primarily the liver, and in the nervous systems. As they accumulate over time, they cause problems with the nerves, hormones and immune system. Birds affected by household spray insecticides containing chlorinated hydrocarbons can become ill within 48 hours. Symptoms include listlessness, side-to-side head movements, head tremors, eyelid blinking, erratic flight and can actually die while airborne.

Strychnine, used in pesticides, is especially lethal for dogs and cats. Signs of poisoning, such as apprehension and stiffness, can appear within minutes of ingestion. Convulsions develop as the poison spreads, with respiratory arrest causing death.

In "Clinical Toxicities of Cats", Veterinarians Clarke Atkins and Roger Johnson, described a case of strychnine poisoning in a dog who had remained indoors for over 12 hours. The source of the poisoning was discovered to be a meatball, impregnated with the toxin, brought in by the family cat who decided it was not edible. Unfortunately the dog did not share that opinion and consumed part of it.

Birds also, can become a casualty of strychnine poisoning, especially if they eat seed laced with it, (sometimes used as mice poison). Symptoms indicated are paralysis and respiratory failure.

Arsenic, which is used in insecticides, herbicides, ant poisons, snail bait, paints and some drugs can cause acute poisoning. The animal can exhibit severe gastroenteritis, depression, colic, anorexia, extreme weakness and death. Cats can exhibit symptoms within 30 minutes of ingesting larger doses and can die within seven hours. Birds show signs of ruffled feathers, drooping wings, anorexia, and regurgitation.

Pyrethrum (from chrysanthemum flowers) is a non-toxic insecticide and used as a flea repellant. Safe in its natural state, reactions are normally limited to salivation because of its bitter taste, although it can be harmful to frogs and reptiles. Many products contain chemical additives which are dangerous and can cause problems for dogs and cats; hypersalivation, vomiting, diarrhea, mild tremors, hyperexcitability or depression and seizures. These symptoms usually last for up to 3 days unless the animal is re-exposed. Be careful when buying pyrethrins and only use natural safe pyrethrum powders.

Rotenone, touted as semi-toxic, is derived from the derris plant. If ingested by a cat it may cause nausea and vomiting and in the long term can promote liver damage. Sabadilla also considered less toxic, comes from the seeds of the South American lily, and is harmful to bees and humans who come in direct contact with it. How safe can it be for pets who walk or roll in plants treated with this substance? Nicotine is sometimes applied instead of toxic pesticides, but this can be deadly to pets, birds and fish. Just because an insecticide is labeled non-toxic does not mean it is safe for your pet.

NON-TOXIC PEST CONTROL METHODS

IPM, Integrated Pest Management, is a methodology whereby insects are controlled through biological and other means which are environmentally friendly. They try to use as many non-toxic applications as possible, for instance a botanical insecticide extracted from the seeds of the Neem tree in Southeast Asia which repels armyworms, aphids and Japanese beetles. Horticultural oils such as Sunspray Oil works by smothering insects instead of poisoning them.

In your vegetable garden, try companion planting. Certain bugs will not eat carrots if they grow next to tomatoes which they don't like. (My favorite garden book is "Carrots Love Tomatoes"). Also strengthen your plants through proper feeding of kelp, compost and minerals. Strong plants are less likely to attract predators. Organic gardeners never use pesticides. More and more farmers are turning to organic methods, not because they are purists, but because pesticides don't work anymore. Bugs have developed such a strong resistance to pesticides that the quantity of toxins needed for control costs more than the farmer can afford. Numerous books have been written on the subject and it would be wise to do your own investigation.

If you despise mosquitos, instead of harmful bug sprays, use citronella-based repellents usually found in health food stores. Install bird houses to attract purple martins, or bat houses to encourage bat colonies. Both will devastate mosquito populations. Bats are beneficial creatures and should not be treated as predators.

Ants and roaches can be repelled by using Lemon Grass and also borates. The latter must be used carefully as only one teaspoon can kill a pet. Tea tree oil and eucalyptus oil have been thought to be a pest repellent, but only use in diluted form as concentrated amounts may cause near fatal poisonings. Rosemary, bay leaves or citronella work well to keep bugs away if you are enjoying an evening on the back porch. Exterminating termites can be successful using the safe "Heatwave" system which "cooks" the wood to temperatures of 130 degrees and kills the inhabitants.

RAT POISON HAZARDS

It should be obvious that if rodent bait kills rats, then it is extremely hazardous if eaten by your pet. Remember some pet haters will purposely put this toxin out as a poison. If you notice any one of the following symptoms in your pet, contact a vet immediately: nervousness, restlessness, muscle rigidity, convulsions, profuse salivation, nausea or watery diarrhea. Medical attention may not be successful in preventing permanent damage or death, therefore the best preventative method is to know your pet's "haunts" and patrol them often for poisons.

LETHAL FLEA KILLERS

All people hate fleas and will do anything to keep them away. A best seller in insect repellent is N,N-diethyl-m-toluamide (DEET). This substance can also be found in some flea repellents. We know that certain symptoms can arise with repeated use on our pets, and have even heard that cats 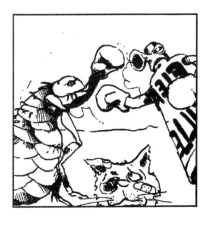 continually given flea baths containing DEET, have died.

It is estimated that 22% of the general population in the

U.S. is exposed yearly to DEET-based products, especially as a mosquito repellant. This substance can penetrate the skin of Guinea pigs within 6 hours and may cause problems with the central nervous system. Cats and dogs may develop tremors, vomiting, excitation and seizures. Human children can also be affected through exposure, exhibiting signs of lethargy, behavioral changes, abnormal movements, seizures and coma as well as chemical burns to sensitive skin. Remember this when considering purchasing a product containing DEET and choose a less toxic alternative.

Commercial flea collars contain chemicals that supposedly kill the pests, but if your pet is like mine, fleas always hop over the collars and end up on your pet's face. They may not be as affective at killing the fleas as they are with inflicting your pet with permanent health damage. Would you consciously decide to wear toxic pesticides around your neck if you knew they caused cancer? If not, why are you making your pet suffer?

Chemical flea collars can pose a real threat to small animals. Some contain DDVP, which is more toxic to the parasites than they are to dogs, but sensitive animals can exhibit excessive salivation, watery diarrhea, and respiratory difficulties. The smaller the animal the greater the risk as the constant breathing of these toxic fumes can cause permanent damage to internal organs. Dichlorvos-impregnated flea collars may cause contact dermatitis in some pets.

Most chemical flea collars come with explicit warnings about their toxicity for humans: dust from this collar is harmful if swallowed, and will cause eye problems; if not removed from pets during baths, make sure shampoo contaminated with collar dust does not get in eyes; follow disposal directions properly. With all these considerations, choose only natural, non-toxic flea collars.

In an effort to rid our homes of fleas, we subject ourselves and our pets to permanent health risk from foggers (bombs). In big letters on the "bomb" box, warnings indicate fumes are not to be inhaled, and mist is not to be inhaled or absorbed through the skin. Food and cooking surfaces are to be covered, vehicles removed from garages and fish aquariums and plants covered prior to use. People and pets are to vacate the home during use, but allowed to return after the fumes have settled.

Active-ingredients may include DDVP, propoxur, diazinon and carbaryl, all nerve poisons toxic to pets and humans. Since these pesticides have long half-lives, their residue does not go away. It remains in furnishings, carpets, drapes, wood...all things your pet comes in contact with. The sad outcome to this toxic assault on your house is that the fleas don't stay away and repeated "bombings" are necessary, doubling and tripling the chance for sickness. Many people develop allergies within their homes after fumigation, some which last as long as they live in the house. These toxins cannot be removed unless the house is gutted, therefore the only cure for the symptoms is to move.

SAFE FLEA CONTROL METHODS

There are non hazardous flea collars and shampoos that use pennyroyal, eucalyptus, cedar and citronella as "insecticides". Some animals may exhibit a salivation reaction to some of these herbs and may not be able to wear them. As an alternative, sprinkle nutritional yeast (not Brewers Yeast, which can cause skin problems, allergies or vomiting), in their food once a day and lo and behold...no more fleas. It seems the ingredients in yeast causes a certain odor to be produced in the skin. This makes the pet unappetizing to fleas and ticks. Garlic and sulfur (a key mineral element) can do the same, causing a reaction which emits hydrogen sulfide on the surface of the skin, making it unappetizing to fleas.

Substitutions for lethal whole-house flea treatments can be as easy as baking them out. After removing living things, turn the heat as high as it will go and leave the house. The fleas will die from the heat. Carpet and bedding sprays containing citronella, eucalyptus and lemon grass 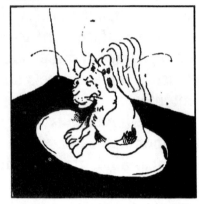 oils do a much better job than chemical foggers and sprays. They will normally not make you or your pet sick. Beware of solutions containing pennyroyal or citrus extracts as they can be harmful to animals, especially cats. Some flea powders containing pyrethrum may be toxic to pets if they contain additives. Only natural pyrethrum products are safe. Don't sprinkle borate carpet treatments on your floors because pets become sick when they lick it off their paws.

Outdoors you may try flea-eating nematodes, sprinkled in areas where you pet lies down. They need moisture to survive, therefore keep those areas damp. There are also "flea birth control hormones" methoprene and fenoxycarb, that do not affect mammals. They prevent flea eggs and larvae from maturing into adults and are available in sprays and flea collars. Of course, diligence may be the best flea treatment for your pet. If adding nutritional yeast to your pet's diet works, you won't have to bother with any other removal method. Flea combs and non-toxic flea sprays can tackle the problem when you groom your pet (if you have the time). The last word is to throw out all your toxic flea repellents and sprays as they compromise your health. Fumes may leak during storage, be absorbed by your skin and inhaled during application.

KILLING OUR PETS
WITH CLEANLINESS

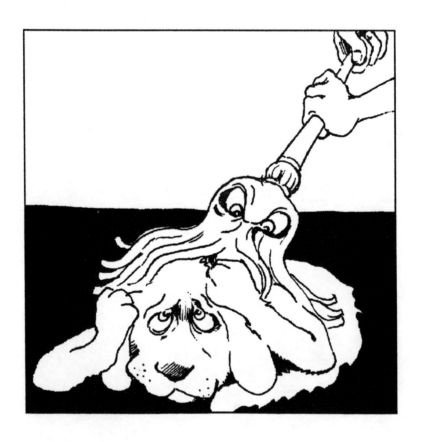

Many of us have an obsession with keeping our living space clean. Our cupboards are filled with floor cleaners, wall cleaners, air fresheners, carpet cleaners and deodorizers, tile cleaners, waxes, abrasives, spot removers, bleaches, stain resistant sprays, soaps and drain cleaners. None of the product manufacturers recommend ingesting them through the mouth or eyes. Warnings on many labels instruct us to use them only in a well-ventilated place. Does this mean you shouldn't breathe them either? You may not be able to determine how toxic a substance is because normally ingredients are not listed, or if they are, we have no idea what all those big words mean. People clean and clean, and polish and polish, and go to work knowing their house shines, but have they left their pets inside to get poisoned?

Aerosols are known to cause spiratory stress and asthma in people. Why wouldn't they also affect pets with the same affliction? Americans pour more than 32 million pounds of household cleaning products down the drain each day. These substances go into our water system, and if not properly filtered, can come back to haunt us and our pets in drinking water. Natural and biodegradable alternatives are the answer.

Also dangerous to pets are Nonstick cooking pans, office and artist products. Glues, whiteout, toners, pens, paint, solvents, crayons, clay, etc. can all cause illness if eaten or licked by your dog or cat. Parents are careful to teach children not to put anything other than food in their mouths. Unfortunately, animals rarely learn that lesson and therefore get sick from "harmless" materials not put out of their reach. Nonstick pans when heated to high temperatures (above 530 degrees F) release polytetra-fluoroethylene gas which is toxic if inhaled by birds. Most cooking temperatures are below this but if you forget and overheat the pan, it could kill your bird.

Just like pesticides, the chemicals in many household cleaners can cause genetic damage in our pets. Most animal studies have determined that cancer is evident with toxic levels of chemical ingestion. Only recently have they begun to study the reproductive effects of these contaminants. Called "hormonal" pollutants, breakdown products of common detergents have been indicated in causing increased levels of female estrogen in male animals.

This can have widespread implications, and although you may not notice it in your altered dog or cat, it can be the demise of many species of wildlife. Our lifestyles do have far-reaching effects and what we put down our sink or release into the air could eventually kill backyard wildlife visitors. Be responsible and consider all implications of your actions when you go shopping for household products.

SYMPTOMS OF
CLEANING PRODUCT POISONING

VOMITING/DIARRHEA
BURNS OF MOUTH AND ESOPHAGUS
HYPER-SALIVATION
MUSCLE WEAKNESS
CENTRAL NERVOUS SYSTEM DEPRESSION
SEIZURES
SLOW RESPIRATION
CORNEAL DAMAGE
HYPERTHERMIA
ANXIETY
COLIC
RESTLESSNESS

CATS

ABOVE PLUS
HAIR LOSS
SKIN ULCERATIONS
HYPERACTIVITY
PANTING
SHOCK
CARDIAC ARRHYTHMIA
COMA
DEATH

CLEANING PRODUCT RISKS

Pets are more susceptible to hazardous cleaning products because they spend most of their lives on the floor where fumes are the strongest. Cats may walk over freshly washed or waxed floors and then lick the cleaner off their paws. Animals can roll on the carpet which is impregnated with anti-flea dust, carpet freshener or spot cleaners and pick up toxins in their fur. Aerosol sprays don't do much for their health either especially if they already have respiratory problems.

Fumes left over from cleaning applications can linger in the home for long periods of time, especially when the windows are closed during the heating or air conditioning seasons. Also dangerous are those nice smelling air fresheners we all are fanatical about buying. Laden with chemicals, they are not to be eaten, therefore why breathe them? Pets have no choice. They are in a toxic gas chamber that you have created.

Concerns about sickness from cleaning products constituted 4% of all calls to the Illinois Animal Poison Information Center in 1987. These included general cleaners, toilet cleaners, bleaches, corrosives, laundry products, disinfectants, carpet products, bath and tile cleaners, floor and wall cleaners, dish washing detergents and industrial cleaners. Approximately 85% of all the calls involved accidental exposure within the home, mostly from oral ingestion. Dogs seemed to be more likely to be exposed than cats because they will put just about anything in their mouth.

SOAP AND LAUNDRY PRODUCT DANGERS

Commercial bar soaps provide the most common source of toxicity. They can cause vomiting and diarrhea possibly because of the essential oils and fragrances used, but they are low in toxicity.

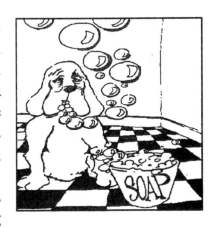

Nonionic synthetic detergents found in hand dish washing liquids and shampoos include alkyl ethoxylate, alkyl phenoxy polyethoxy ethanols, and polyethylene glycol stearate. Animals exposed to these agents will also exhibit vomiting and diarrhea, disrupting their electrolyte balance.

Anionic detergents most normally found in laundry products are alkyl sodium sulfates, alkyl sodium sulfonates, dioctyl sodium sulfosuccinate, sodium lauryl sulfate, tetra-proplylene benzene sulfonate and linear alkyl benzene sulfonates. You may not be able to pronounce these words, but look at the labels on your cleaning products and many will be listed.

The skin, unless broken, is a good barrier to any detergents. If ingested, they are able to be metabolized by the liver and excreted in urine, although cases have been reported of impaired liver function due to concentrations of detergent in the blood. Animals can still exhibit symptoms like diarrhea and vomiting and if the substance gets into their eyes, damage can occur. It is responsible to use the least toxic biodegradable soap products that are available. They will have the least harmful effect on your pet.

Fabric softeners, germicides and sanitizers can burn your

pet's mouth and esophagus, damage mucous membranes, cause hyper-salivation, vomiting, muscle weakness, central nervous system depression and seizures, coma and death. Cats can exhibit hair loss and skin ulcerations and all animals can receive corneal damage if these poisons contact their eyes.

DEADLY DISINFECTANT CLEANERS

Disinfectant cleaners usually have more than one chemical in them, such as cresol, phenol, formaldehyde, ammonia, chlorine and ethanol. Because of the chemical reactions, they can have a more toxic effect. Cats are more susceptible to products containing phenols and if ingested can cause burns 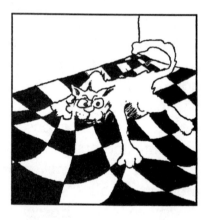 of the mouth and esophagus, vomiting, hyper-salivation, apprehension, hyperactivity and panting. Their toxicity can progress to include shock, cardiac arrhythmias and coma.

Pine oil can also affect cats in a similar manner. If a cat has lapped up this substance they will develop a pine smelling breath and if they drank enough pine oil can die within 12 hours.

Bleaches can cause the same symptoms although the animal may have "bleach (chlorine)" breath which may not cause as rapid demise as pine oil. Inhalation of fumes from bleach powders can cause coughing and retching. Mixing chlorine bleach with ammonia or vinegar can produce chloramine fumes which are quite toxic. Non-chlorine bleach products are generally low toxicity and cause only gastritis. Non-chlorine bleaches are safer, but should still be kept away from animals. Keep all cleaners out of your dog's reach as they may chew open the containers. Make sure any spills are completely wiped up to prevent your pet from lapping up the poison or licking it off their fur.

"NON-TOXIC" CITRUS CLEANERS

Many non-toxic cleaners are based on citrus oils. These are by far safer than chemical detergents. Pet shampoos are normally not a concern because they contain a well diluted form of citrus, but undiluted concentrates of citrus, containing D-limonene, linalool found in food additives, or dog and cat flea sprays can be dangerous. Crude citrus oil extract may be particularly toxic to cats. If exposed to undiluted concentrations of these substances cats can exhibit hyper-salivation and, depending on the level of exposure, can get muscle tremors (shivering), fall over and develop hypothermia (decrease in body temperature). Most cats recover although occasionally death can occur if the animal becomes totally immersed in the liquid, (such as is instructed on some flea dips containers). To be safe follow the manufacturer's recommendations for dilution and store out of reach of pets. Most pet shampoos and skin products containing a highly diluted form of citrus are safe to animals. Read labels carefully or contact the manufacturer if you are concerned.

GARAGE AND BASEMENT POISONS

Almost anything you use for heavy cleaning, painting or servicing your car, can be toxic to animals. A common garage poison is anti-freeze (ethylene glycol). If your radiator is leaking or someone changes the anti-freeze, make sure you clean up any spills completely. Anti-freeze contains a variety of elements in addition to ethylene glycol, such as gasoline, copper, zinc and lead.

Never pour anti-freeze into a stream or onto the ground as it is a sweet-tasting liquid and very attractive to animals, who love to lap it up. Within one-half hour to an hour, following ingestion of a toxic dose, dogs can show signs of anxiety, nausea and depression which progress to a comatose state and death in 6 to 18 hours. It commonly causes cardiac failure and brain damage in household pets who drink it. If smaller amounts are ingested, the animal may vomit and reduce the concentration of the chemical, but his life span may still be shortened to two weeks.

Searching further in the garage we find all sorts of animal "poisons" such as creosol, naphthalene (moth balls), paraffin, phenol, toluene, xylene, hexachlorophene (germicidal soap) and pine tar. Animals can exhibit excessive salivation, weakness, convulsions, hypothermia, paralysis and death from contact with these substances. These are known carcinogens in humans and may be linked to the ever increasing cancer cases seen by veterinarians.

Kerosene and fuel oil are highly toxic, producing gastroenteritis, circulatory collapse, depression, convulsions and coma. Turpentine not only can be poisonous when ingested, but can affect animals through the skin. It manifests nausea, colic, restlessness, coma and death due to respiratory failure.

Chances of fumes from these stored toxins affecting animals is slight as they don't spend much time in a closed garage. Illness, contracted from ingestion caused by spills or leaky containers is more likely. Remember for your pet's (and your children's) safety, keep all garage toxins out of their reach and tightly closed. Clean up after usage and dispose of containers, brushes and rags in properly sealed containers.

PRODUCT SUBSTITUTES FOR TOXIC CLEANERS

Some less toxic cleaners can still have an adverse effect on our pets, but they are less hazardous than their chemical counterparts. These still should be handled with care, stored properly and allowed to dry before allowing your pets to come in contact with them.

Vinegar works well instead of ammonia. Borax, lemon juice, dried kelp, coconut-oil derivatives, baking soda and salt can be used in combinations as they are found in natural cleaning products. Non-chlorine bleaches are preferred. A combination of white vinegar, lemon juice and olive oil can act as furniture polish. Vinegar can be used as a fabric softener, and for silver polish you can use salt water and baking soda in an aluminum pot.

Borax, baking soda, white vinegar and lemon juice are all good spot removers. Baking soda and cornstarch are great carpet fresheners. Lemon grass or cinnamon sticks can be used as natural air fresheners or use citrus/vegetable extract evaporators. Alternatives to mothballs are cedar shavings, lemon grass, lavender, and rosemary. Putting clothes in the dryer or freezer will cook or freeze the larvae.

Zeolites, crushed porous rocks, are safe deodorizers for litter boxes, pet houses and runs. They also eliminate urine odor from carpets and can be used in place of tomatoes for removing skunk odor on your dog. Non-toxic paints, strippers and solvents are widely available from catalogs, eco-stores and some retail paint outlets. Low VOC paints are less toxic if inhaled, but still can be lethal if your pet drinks them. Please be responsible and keep all cleaning and decorating products away from your pets.

CARBON MONOXIDE
POISONING

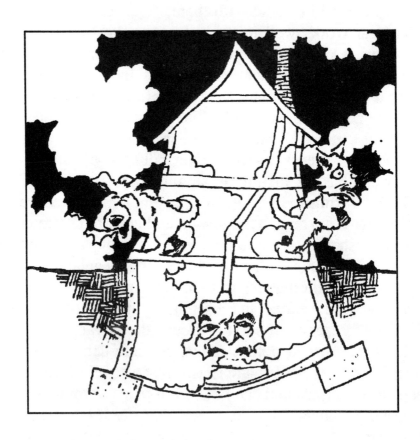

No pet owners ever want to come home and find their dog, cat, or bird dead, especially when they weren't sick. Carbon monoxide (CO) can put them to sleep permanently without anything being disturbed. Pet owners sometimes are in a quandary as to what took their animal's life. Carbon monoxide kills people too, therefore if your pet has died in the house unexpectedly, you had better investigate CO poisoning because you may be next. Better yet, take this chapter seriously and prevent this deadly gas from ever making you or your pet a statistic.

SYMPTOMS OF
CARBON MONOXIDE POISONING

SHORTNESS OF BREATH

HYPER-IRRITABILITY

NAUSEA

VOMITING

CONFUSION

COLLAPSE

CONVULSIONS

COMA

DEATH

CARBON MONOXIDE (CO) DEFINITION

Carbon Monoxide is a colorless, odorless gas that interferes with the delivery of oxygen to cells in the body. Carbon Dioxide is a relatively harmless gas that can be found, for example, in the bubbles in soft drinks. It should not be confused with dangerous carbon monoxide.

CO SOURCES

CO can be found any place where combustion appliances are in use. The most common risk area in the home is in closed garages, if automobiles are left running. Other sources can be furnaces, gas appliances, fireplaces, gas or kerosene space heaters, and charcoal grills used indoors.

One major danger to pets is carbon monoxide which enters the home through the fireplace or chimney. This usually happens because houses that have been built to the new insulation standards have few air leaks. Because of this, the furnace does not get the air it needs to operate properly. It creates negative pressure sucking fumes from the furnace exhaust pipe located in or near the fireplace chimney into the home. This can kill your pet if left at home alone.

If your home is heated by a forced hot air furnace, leaks may cause gas to spread into the house more quickly through the hot air ducting. Some paint removers and solvents containing methylenechloride can evaporate fumes and change to CO. Home fireplaces can emit CO if they are not burning completely and the flues may be clogged or improperly installed.

Chances are that if your home is heated electrically you have an electric water heater and your appliances are all electric, the probabilities for carbon monoxide poisoning may be non-existent. If you have a fireplace or woodstove, you still may have a problem, it would be advisable to have a carbon monoxide detector on hand,

You should also be wary of running your car in an attached garage, and make sure you don't barbecue indoors or use gas or kerosene space heaters to augment your electric heat unless they are working properly and are used in a well ventilated place.

People have the chance to leave the house during the day and unless the carbon monoxide is at high concentrations, the pet owners might not be affected, but they could display some symptoms such as sniffles, fatigue, and difficulty concentrating while in the house. If these symptoms clear up when they go outside, suspect carbon monoxide and never leave your pet at home until you have absolutely determined that CO levels are safe. This can be easily accomplished by installing a CO detector.

KEY SOURCES OF CO:

Gas/Oil furnaces, Space Heaters, Gas stoves, Wood stoves, Fireplaces, Gas Clothes Dryers, Cooking grills used indoors, Automobile exhaust.

SYMPTOMS OF CO POISONING

Tests have shown animals have been affected by CO as follows:

COHb= Carboxyhemoglobin (% of carbon monoxide in blood)

10% COHb	no signs
10-20% COHb	shortness of breath during moderate exercise
30% COHb	hyper-irritability, nausea, vomiting
40% COHb	confusion, collapse, coma
50-60 COHb	respiratory failure, coma, convulsions
60-70 COHb	coma,convulsions,depressed heart action,death
70-80 COHb	death within hours
80-90 COHb	death in less than an hour
90+ COHb	death in minutes

Carbon monoxide replaces normal oxygen-carrying hemoglobin in the blood with carboxyhemoglobin (COHb), a compound that prevents life-supporting oxygen from reaching the heart, brain and other body organs.

Carbon Monoxide may also cause permanent brain damage, which, in humans, has been associated with personality changes and loss in memory. Even at low levels of carbon monoxide birds can die if their cages are kept close to faulty gas stoves and heaters.

In humans. symptoms of CO poisoning can cause flu-like symptoms, dizziness, headaches and nausea, confusion, disorientation and fatigue. Exposure to high concentrations of CO for as little as two hours can result in unconsciousness and death. If you notice any of these symptoms, check your CO detector and don't leave your pet alone until the problem is fixed.

Statistics show that nearly 300 human deaths per year are caused by non fire related carbon monoxide poisoning, from fuel-burning appliances. One can only guess how many pets succumbed. Winter months are especially dangerous as closed windows trap lethal dosages of this gas and usually claim its victims while they sleep. If you think carbon monoxide is affecting your pet, it may also be affecting you.

Ask yourself the following questions:

-Do you feel sleepy, have headaches, dizziness, nausea?
-Do you have watery eyes, nose or throat irritation without having a cold or other known illness?
-Do the symptoms only occur in your house or office?
-Do they go away after you have left for awhile?
-Does anyone else in the house gets symptoms?
-Have you had more cases of flu lately?

-Are your symptoms getting worse?

-Do you have any combustion appliances in your home or office?

If your answer to any of these questions is YES, then maybe your pet is also being affected. This is the one major source of poisoning where you can be affected as well as your pet, but at least <u>you</u> can verbalize your symptoms and take action before something fatal happens.

DETECTION OF CARBON MONOXIDE LEVELS IN PETS

A veterinarian can establish the diagnosis of CO by means of a blood test that measures the blood level of CO combined with hemoglobin. Because CO leaves the blood slowly, this test can pinpoint the problem even if the blood specimen is taken 1 or 2 hours after you have left the suspected environment. The results can tell whether CO is affecting your pet's health. If the gas is found in their body, then you should immediately rectify the problem at the source in your home and prevent carbon monoxide from poisoning your family.

IMMEDIATE SOLUTIONS

.If you suspect your pet's symptoms are attributed to carbon monoxide, get fresh air immediately by opening windows and doors, shutting off appliances, and going outdoors.

.Contact a veterinarian immediately and tell him you suspect this poisoning.

.Examine yourself for symptoms. If any of your symptoms occur only while you are in the house or for a period of time afterwards, suspect CO as the culprit if you have any combustion appliances operating.

SOLUTIONS TO PROTECT OUR PETS FROM CO POISONING

A simple inexpensive carbon monoxide detector test kit provides a colormetric disk which you can affix to any area in the home. The disk will change color if CO is present, and the time it takes to turn color can indicate how severe the levels of concentration are. For example, on a colormetric detector it takes 15-45 minutes for 100 parts per million of CO to indicate a problem. At 600 ppm it only takes 1-2 minutes. Indicators may have faster reaction time if the weather is damp and slower when dry. Any indication is cause for alarm.

It is best to install the colormetric detectors in several rooms and check them several times per day to see if any change has taken place. People may use the test, determine that their home is safe one day, and not check again. Appliances can have faulty systems that go all of a sudden, therefore constant monitoring is prudent. A more reliable alternative is the automatic electrically operated CO detectors which sound an alarm if the gas is present. They need no daily checking. You should install one of these units on each floor of your house. Many states are considering legislation that would make them mandatory in certain types of housing and are similar to the automatic smoke alarms. The city of Chicago has implemented a program for CO detector requirements.

Proper ventilation is essential to diluting any hazards from combustion appliances. Opening a window and running exhaust fans can help, but your heating bills will go up. Heat recovery ventilators (installations that bring fresh air into the home while exhausting the stale air) can do the job with minimal heat loss, but installation is difficult unless you are building a new structure or have an existing forced hot air system.

The most important part of heating season readiness is to have your service person clean your furnace and make sure the flame is adjusted to maintain a clean burn. Have the heat box checked for cracks and repaired, and make sure there is an adequate air supply to and around the furnace, preferably ducting air intake from outside the house.

Clean the flue yourself if maintenance personnel are not available and make sure you change any furnace filter frequently. Hire maintenance personnel to clean any forced hot air ducts you may have prior to the heat being turned on.

Make sure the flame on your furnace or hot water heater is blue. Yellow flames indicates that the burner must be adjusted. The yellow color is due to carbon in the flame which produces carbon monoxide. If you smell fuel, suspect a problem and call maintenance.

Furnaces made after 1982 have a pilot light safety system called an oxygen depletion sensor (ODS), which shuts off the heater when there is not enough fresh air to have an effective burn. Consider buying gas appliances that have electronic ignitions as they eliminate the continuous low-level pollutants from pilot lights. No furnace is guaranteed to prevent carbon monoxide from entering the house, but with proper maintenance and upkeep, they should work as designed and not pose a hazard.

During the time the heater is on, check the flame frequently to assure complete burn, make sure that all panels and grills are in place and that the fan door be closed when the furnace is operating.

Make sure flue is open for either wood or gas fireplaces

and clean the flue and chimney each fall. As in fire prevention, make sure the fire is out before you go to sleep. Maintain good ventilation whenever a woodstove or fire-place is in operation.

If you have a kerosene or other space heater fueled by a combustible material, make sure that you have adequate ventilation. This not only keeps the unit burning efficiently (less CO emitted) but also protects you from harmful concentrations of any gas buildup. You should always use a carbon monoxide detector when using these supplemental heaters.

Never run your car in a closed garage, especially if it is attached to the house. Fumes from the exhaust can be sucked into the home and can remain for a period of time, especially if the home is well insulated. Never use outdoor barbecue grills in a closed room unless they are vented to the outside. Many people and pets have died due to carbon monoxide from using charcoal grills indoors in inclement weather when the windows are closed.

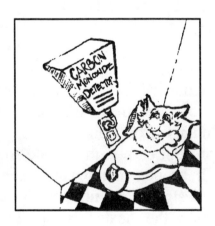

LEAD POISONING

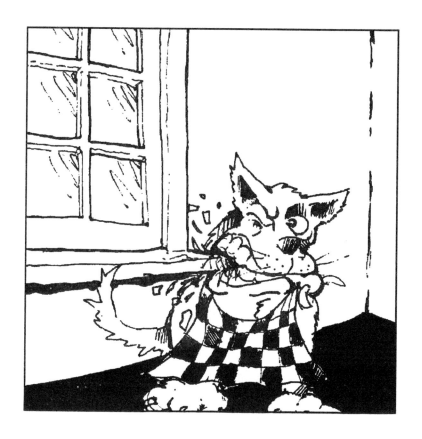

Many veterinarians have diagnosed lead poisoning in animals. Often this comes after the pet owner has disclosed that the animal was chewing on window sills, or that they had recently renovated their home. Unfortunately, most of us inadvertently may cause danger to our trusting pets. As we try to make our homes more comfortable, we sand and scrape and apply that fresh coat of paint with little regard to the makeup of subsurface materials. During this time, our pets may come to investigate our progress, and get contaminated.

We usually spend a considerable amount of time cleaning up our mess, but if the old paint that we attacked was lead paint, vacuuming is not enough. Our animals walk in this dust, breathe it resulting in a diagnosis of lead poisoning by the vet. This hazard is quite common in older homes. In more recently built houses, lead paint isn't used, but pets can still develop some health symptoms by ingesting dust from most commercial chemical-based paints. A good rule of thumb is to keep all animals away from any work areas during renovation and use proper clean-up methods. If you have an older home, please purchase a lead paint test kit. These are very easy to use. Determining the consistency of paint before you sand will save your family and your pets health.

If you discover that your home lead test reveals a substantial amount of lead paint, you should consider calling a lead remediation company for advice. As lead paint can have lasting effects on pets and children, it is imperative that you analyze your home and do a self test if you suspect any lead paint.

SYMPTOMS OF LEAD POISONING

DOGS

COLIC
ANEXORIA
VOMITING
DIARRHEA
RESTLESSNESS
WHINING
GROWLING
CHOMPING OF JAWS
RUNNING IN ALL DIRECTIONS
KIDNEY PROBLEMS
REPRODUCTIVE DISORDERS

CATS

GASTRIC UPSET
HYSTERIA
NEUROLOGICAL SYMPTOMS
CONVULSIONS
KIDNEY PROBLEMS
REPRODUCTIVE DISORDERS

BIRDS

NERVOUS SYSTEM MALFUNCTIONS
MUSCLE SPASMS

LEAD

Lead is found as an ore in its natural state in the earth's crust. Because it is durable, resists corrosion, and has a low melting point, etc..., lead is indispensable in many industries. It has been used in gasoline, paint, solder, water pipes, housewares, crystal, pottery, children's toys, and batteries.

LEAD LOCATIONS

The main source of lead poisoning is from lead paint, which was outlawed in 1978. This paint is typically found on kitchen and bathroom walls and doors, windows and woodwork of pre-1950 homes. If this paint has deteriorated, the pulverized lead dust will be released into the air. If it is on windows and sills the repeated opening of windows can cause further chipping of the paint with the residual dust being cast into the interior air. Pets can be affected by breathing lead dust from paint renovation. Cats may be poisoned after lying on driveways treated with ash from lead smelters and then licking the substance off their fur.

Other sources of lead can be crystal, pottery, older food storage cans, toys and water. Plumbing can contain lead solder or lead pipes. Lead solder can combine with copper pipes creating galvanic corrosion between the two metals and release relatively large amounts of lead into the water. Pets which drink contaminated water can become adversely affected.

Recent regulations from the 1988 amendments to the Safe Drinking Water Act, have reduced the maximum amount of lead in solder used for water pipes to 2%. Faucets can also contain lead, since the insides of most faucets are made of brass, an alloy of copper, zinc and other metallic substances. It is estimated that 17% of the nation's homes have faucets leaking high amounts of lead.

A story was told about a cat who got lead poisoning by sitting on a windowsill next to an area that had a great source of automobile fumes, when lead was still an ingredient in gasoline. Birds pecking at lead ceramics, putty, paint on their cages and lead weights (used as curtain weights), can affect their nervous system and muscles. Guinea Pigs have a high tolerance to the lead in printing ink from newspapers lining their cages and have not had adverse reactions.

LEAD DANGERS FOR YOUNG ANIMALS

Just as in children, young animals' growing bodies are forming bones. Lead is absorbed and stored in the same way as calcium because the body cannot distinguish the difference. This will lead to future problems such as neurological symptoms, kidney and reproductive disorders, blindness and death. In young animals up to 90 per cent of lead can be absorbed whereas in adults only 10 per cent.

As harbingers, young dogs seem to give us clues as to impending lead poisoning of young children. Dogs live and eat in the same environment and develop signs of lead poisoning, identifiable long before signs are obvious in children. Any family having a dog diagnosed with lead poisoning should immediately have their children tested. If your house fits the criteria for possibly having lead paint, then you should be familiar with signs of lead poisoning and take action.

RISKS TO DOGS

Dogs are affected by lead poisoning in much greater numbers than cats, probably due to the fact that they chew wood coated with lead paint. Dogs are most affected between two and eight months of age because of constant teething. The exception to this would be in the case of lead poisoning through contaminated drinking water.

LEAD POISONING SYMPTOMS

Cats usually show signs of lead poisoning by gastric upset, hysteria, neurological symptoms and convulsion. Dogs exhibit colic, anorexia, vomiting, diarrhea, restlessness, whining and groaning, chomping of the jaws, running in every direction, indiscriminate biting, blindness and convulsions. Lead poisoning in dogs can be mis-diagnosed as canine distemper.

Identification and treatment is best left to a veterinarian who will determine the proper chelation therapy. Under this treatment animals may improve in 24 to 48 hours.

LEAD PAINT

The Environmental Protection Agency estimates that two-thirds of the homes in the U.S. built before 1940 had lead paint (containing up to 50% lead) in them. From 1940-1960 one-third had lead paint and less than one-third since 1960. Lead paint produced after the 1940's reportedly had lower concentrations than earlier lead-based paint. It is estimated that about three million tons of lead remain in fifty-seven million occupied private housing units built before 1980. Yours could be one of them.

In 1978 the Consumer Product Safety Commission banned lead paint, typically found on kitchen and bathroom walls in older homes (before 1950), on doors, door trim and window trim. Most of these contaminated surfaces have been painted over, but don't let that give you a false sense of security. As long as these painted areas are kept up, and your animal doesn't chew the surface, you should be safe, but if the paint is chipping or flaking, lead paint and dust could be a problem. If you repaint the lead paint area, be careful not to scrape or sand unless you take proper precautions. Lead chips and lead dust can infect your animals as the residue remains in the air and in cracks on the floor long after you thought you had cleaned them up. Contact your local heath department or lead remediation contractor for proper lead paint treatment.

LEAD IN WATER

It has been reported that the water in as many as 20% of American households contain elevated lead levels. This comes from lead plumbing, lead service pipes, lead water supply pipes, lead in faucets and from lead solder. In some areas, cisterns are still used to store water or act as part of roof collection systems. These cisterns may be constructed with a lead liner or may have lead solder used for construction or repairs and if the water has a relatively low pH, it can dissolve lead in the cistern, and cause it to leach into the water. Lead can come from public water systems, as old lead pipes carry the water from reservoirs or water facilities.

The EPA estimated that as many as thirty million people served by 819 good-sized public water systems, could be drinking water containing unsafe high lead levels. It is a possibility that your faucet is constructed with lead alloys. Newer faucets seem to have the highest concentrations of lead, and it is suspected that one sixth of the nation's homes have faucets leaking high amounts of lead.

If your home has lead pipes or lead solder and hard water, a scale may have built up inside the pipe and protect the water from lead contamination. If, in an effort to reduce the scaling, you add a water softener, the scale will disappear and the soft water will act on the lead to leach it into the water system.

Indoor pets have no choice as the to water they drink. Their humans either give them water or they drink out of the toilet bowl. If this water contains lead from pipes or water sources, the animal will ingest it. Ceramic water dishes can contain lead. If you wish to protect your family and your pet from lead poisoning, purchase a home lead-in-water test kit, which can give you an indication if further professional analysis is necessary to determine how serious the problem is.

Some of the 30 U.S. water systems having the highest lead levels:

CHARLESTON, SOUTH CAROLINA
COLUMBIA, SOUTH CAROLINA
UTICA, NEW YORK
YONKERS, NEW YORK
CAMP LEJEUNE, NORTH CAROLINA

Some of the 10 largest U.S. water systems with high lead levels:

NEW YORK, NEW YORK
PHILADELPHIA, PENNSYLVANIA

NEW YORK, NEW YORK
PHILADELPHIA, PENNSYLVANIA
DETROIT, MICHIGAN
WASHINGTON, D.C.
BOSTON, MASSACHUSETTS
SAN FRANCISCO, CALIFORNIA

COMMON SOURCES OF LEAD CONTAMINATION

Windows, Shutters, Ceilings, Doors, Trim, Shelving, Toys, Walls, Furniture, Floors, Brick, Cabinets, Ceramics, Food Care, Dinnerware, Railings, Stairs, Counters, Concrete, Radiators, Pipes, Lead solder, Dirt, Dust.

LEAD SOLUTIONS

The first step is to determine if your home has lead contamination. You can perform your own lead tests with kits you can buy in hardware stores. These kits give you strips of material impregnated with a substance. When moistened and applied to a surface containing lead paint, these strips will turn pink or red. They can indicate lead paint, lead in dishes, toys, dirt, etc. If lead paint is found then you should hire a professional lead testing company to perform either an x-ray fluorescence analyzer(XRF) test on the walls or determine the extensive lead contaminated area through laboratory testing of samples taken at specified distances. These tests will indicate whether it is necessary to do a complete renovation or just remodeling of certain areas.

If your surfaces have been painted before 1978, the chances are, that lead based paint was used. If extensive areas of lead paint are found, the best corrective method is to replace the surface that is painted. This is best done by a licensed contractor who will take the proper precautions to contain any dust that could remain in the air within the rooms. When removing lead paint, a great amount of dust is put into the air within the home. This dust can be extremely hazardous if inhaled by you, your children and your pets. Licensed remediation contractors have ways, that are approved by the state health offices, of containing the dust. It is advised that you move away from the structure during renovation to avoid contact with the lead dust. This includes taking your pets with you. For a listing of approved lead removal contractors contact your state health office. Never attempt removal yourself.

In order to protect your pet from lead paint which is in good condition, routinely clean the floors, window sills and baseboards with either trisodium phosphate cleaner or phosphate free LFA-11, a detergent developed for lead contaminated dust removal. As with all chemicals, keep pets away until surfaces are dry and fumes have dissipated. Remove carpets if lead dust is suspected. When cleaning carpets with a vacuum, dust may be tossed into the air and inhaled or land on tables, dishes, etc. There is no really safe way to remove lead dust from carpet other than replacement.

Obviously, if you have lead pipes, it would be wise to replace them. If that is not feasible or if lead is coming from your water supply lines, the only solution in is to use point-of-use or whole house filtration. Common effective methods are reverse-osmosis, distillation and solid block & precoat adsorption filters, as well as special filters for heavy metal reduction. If Granulated Activated Carbon filters (GAC) are used by themselves, they may not remove lead. This type of filter media is used in many inexpensive commercial point-of-use filters, and If you are considering purchasing a filter system, please specify you need guarantees that their system will remove lead.

RULES TO KEEP PETS SAFE FROM LEAD POISONING:

.Perform a home lead test if you suspect lead in your house.
.Disclose your concern for lead poisoning with your vet if your animal has unusual symptoms.
.If your vet suspects lead poisoning, have him perform a blood test to confirm the level of poisoning.

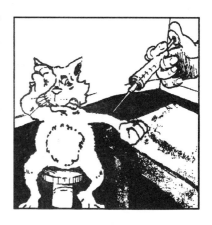

.Keep the house free from dust and wipe areas frequently with soap and water and trisodium phosphate or LFA-11.
.Avoid use of any pet dishes containing lead, and never buy lead soldered canned food.
.Treat wood surfaces with a pet repellent to prevent the animal from chewing them.
.Tape any areas where paint may be chipping, to prevent further paint loss until you can have it removed. Cover any walls with new paint, wallpaper or paneling to prevent pet contact with lead paint.
.If outdoor dirt is suspected or found to be contaminated, try to fence off that area and plant grass to keep the dust down.
.If you know animals have been exposed to lead-contaminated soil area, wash their fur and paws before letting them enter the house.
.If water tests show lead contamination, give pets bottled water or install a water filtration system. Do not give pets

contaminated soil area, wash their fur and paws before letting them enter the house.

.If water tests show lead contamination, give pets bottled water or install a water filtration system. Do not give pets water from the tap. If you must use tap water, let it run for two minutes prior to dispensing it. This may flush out most of the lead from water standing in the pipes.

. Don't let pets chew on children's toys if you suspect they are painted with lead paint.

DANGEROUS PLANTS

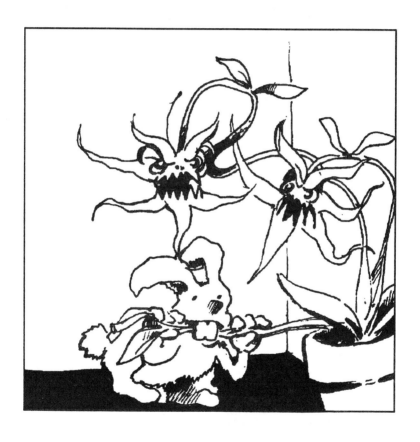

If eaten, common indoor and outdoor plants can cause illness and in extreme cases, death to cats and dogs. Cats may scratch plants and become infected by grooming their claws. Animals also may consume plants as a result of developing illness. If this is the case, you may not be able to determine if the symptom was from the plant.

Plant-based allergic dermatitis or skin rashes may affect humans, but not necessarily pets. If your animal does develop a skin condition, analyze their haunts to determine if a toxic plant may be causing the problem before you call the vet. As in all symptomatic conditions, your pet doctor will better be able to offer treatment if they know the entire story.

Plants that are normally non-toxic to pets can make them sick if they are sprayed with pesticides or fertilizers. If these toxins are applied to a plant poisonous to your pet they may mask or alter adverse clinical signs of illness from the plant itself.

Non-toxic plants can still cause stomach upset in your pet, even if they are not sprayed. Cats normally eat grass for nutrition and to cause vomiting which facilitates the removal of hairballs, Unfortunately for the cat owner, pets usually wait until they come inside to relieve themselves of their stomach distress.

Outdoor pets are at risk, although there is little you can do to monitor your neighbors plantings or the woods behind your house. You can, however, be conscious of your indoor plants and choose varieties that are non-toxic if you suspect your pet "eyes" them hungrily.

SYMPTOMS OF PLANT POISONING

STOMACH UPSET

VOMITING

WATERY EYES AND NOSE

CONVULSIONS

GASTROENTERITIS

DEATH

IRRITATION OF MOUTH AND LIPS

INTERFERENCE WITH BREATHING

TROUBLE SWALLOWING

EXCESS SALIVATION

SYMPTOMS OF PLANT POISONING

Some common plants used in dried flower arrangements are laurel, rhododendron and azalea which can cause watery eyes or nose, vomiting, convulsions and in the case of laurel, death. Hydrangea and bittersweet result in gastroenteritis and the latter can even cause unconsciousness.

Mistletoe may form a lethal appetizer to a dog who eats it. Even Christmas tree needles and the water from the base can cause gastrointestinal stress. Poinsettias may cause vomiting and even death.

Dieffenbachia can produce irritation of the mouth and lips and possibly interference with breathing and swallowing in dogs, cats and birds. Philodendron may cause irritation of mucous membranes, and excessive salivation in cats.

The bulbs of daffodils, narcissus and jonquil cause severe gastroenteritis and hyacinth can cause trembling and convulsions. Bulbs are a favorite treat of dogs who do a lot of digging.

DANGEROUS PLANTS

Toxic plants and seeds are found in homes and workplaces. Dogs and cats occasionally consume various plants or portions thereof such as catnip, in the case of our intoxicated kitties. The following list should alert you to common plants in your area that could cause your pet a trip to the vet.

House Plants:
Daffodil, Poinsettia, Mistletoe, Philodendron, Indian rubber plant, Dieffenbachia

Flowers:
Delphinium, Foxglove, Monkshood, Iris, Lily of the valley, Amaryllis, Morning glory, Daffodil, Easter lily (cats), Tiger lily (cats)

Vegetables:
Rhubarb, Spinach, Tomato vine

Shrubs:
Daphne, Azalea, Rhododendron, Lantana, Holly, Wormwood

Trees:
Oak , Peach , Cherry, Elderberry , Black locust, Apple (seeds), Oleander

Wild plants:
Jack-in-the-pulpit, Moonseed, May apple , Duchmans breeches, Water hemlock, Mushrooms, Buttercup, Nightshade, Poison hemlock, Jimsonweed, Pigweed, Locoweed, Lupine, Halogeton, Poison ivy, Poison oak

LISTING OF TOXIC PLANTS AND THEIR HAZARDS

The National Animal Poison Control Center has a list of the most common plants, both toxic and non-toxic, including associated problems /hazards. To receive this list write the NAPCC, College of Veterinary Medicine, University of Illinois, Urbana, IL 61801

FOR POISON HELP:

If you are in a panic because you think your pet is poisoned and you are unable to get to a veterinarian immediately, there is a group that can provide you with emergency service. The National Animal Poison Control Center, is THE place to go for help. Do not call your human poison control center as they are not well versed in animal treatments.

The National Animal Poison Control Center (NAPCC), a non-profit service of the University of Illinois, is the first animal-oriented poison center in the United States. The NAPCC's phones are answered by licensed veterinarians and board-certified veterinary toxicologists.

They have an extensive collection of individual cases - over 250,000 - involving pesticide, drug, plant, metal and other exposures in food producing and companion animals. This allows them to make specific recommendations for your animals, rather than generalized poison information provided by a human poison control center. There is a charge for their consultations.

If you require information regarding this valuable service. please contact them at 217-333-2053 or write: Dr. Louise M. Cote', NAPCC, U of Illinois College of Veterinary Medicine, 2001 S. Lincoln Ave., Urbana, IL 61801.

WATER CONTAMINATION

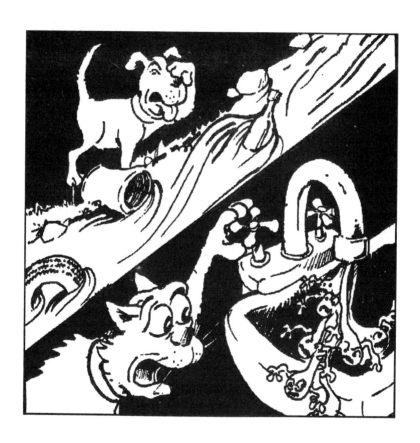

Water is one of the keys to life and if it's polluted, that life may be compromised. Most pets depend on their owners to supply them with fresh water and what do we do...give them a clear liquid with chlorine, fluoride, nitrates, lead, arsenic, pesticides, mercury and hundreds of other pollutants in it.

Water has the ability to dissolve just about all substances that it comes in contact with. These dissolved solids can appear in water as suspended matter or biologicals. When these foreign substances appear in our drinking and bathing water, they can pose health risks.

Today we constantly are warned not to eat fish that may be contaminated with mercury, or shellfish that feed near industrial effluent. Every now and then the newspapers are full of articles about bacteria in drinking waters making whole neighborhoods sick. Water treatment facilities have been created to help clear up the water that flows to our taps, but many are under funded and lack the proper equipment to do the job properly.

Even if you don't live on city water systems, your well can be contaminated from agricultural run-off and industrial ground pollution. Pets can contract many of the same illness as people from drinking contaminated water. For example, some of the following statistics apply to humans, but it may be that a number of pets also get sick from drinking the same water.

-One in six people drink water with excessive amounts of lead in it.

-Microbes in tap water may be responsible for 1 in 3 cases of gastro-intestinal illness.

-The EPA states that in Ohio's 88 counties, death rates for bladder and stomach cancer were more prevalent where drinking water was taken from rivers and lakes than from wells.

-The Natural Resources Defense Council claims that more than 350,000 people drink water with arsenic levels above the federal limit, which has been criticized as being much too lenient.

Animals may be somewhat impervious to biological contamination as they do not seem to become ill every time they drink from a stream or muddy puddle, but chemical contamination may be creating long term chronic sickness. We will address some of the water pollution hazards to humans assuming that animals may be at risk from these same contaminants.

It is essential that our pets drink clean water and it is necessary that they maintain a proper mineral balance. The pet owner's responsibility lies in having the water tested. If adverse contaminants are found, install a water filter and if necessary, add back the minerals. Wild animals drink water from open streams and lakes. This may be hazardous to their health as pollution, acid raid, agricultural runoff and industrial spills can make a toxic cocktail for them. We can do our part by helping to police the waterways and supporting environmental organizations, but we can also stop pollution at home by living non-toxically.

SYMPTOMS FROM
WATER POLLUTION

GASTRIC DISTRESS

CANCER

NEUROLOGICAL SYMPTOMS

ANOREXIA

RESTLESSNESS

DISTEMPER-LIKE SYMPTOMS (DOGS)

DENTAL FLUOROSIS

ECZEMA

STOMACH UPSET

POLLUTANTS IN CITY WATER

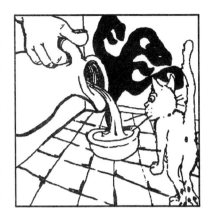

About half the nation's drinking water comes from ground water "aquifers" 20 to 1,000 feet beneath the surface. They are porous formations consisting of layers of sand, gravel or rock and contain areas that allow water to collect above non-porous layers of bedrock. This subsurface water moves very slowly, sometimes as little as three feet per year. Without sun or oxygen to cleanse it, contamination can compound the problem.

Pollutants that leach through surface ground to the aquifers can build to dangerous levels. When these water sources are tapped for drinking and bathing usage, health hazards become a reality. Contamination of surface waters is all too common and when those sources are used for municipal water systems, similar health implications arise.

Landfills can hold over 200 substances, including numerous chemical compounds and with 16,000 dumps in use in the US, potentially 8 million people and pets could be affected when those substances leak out. There are about 2.3 million gasoline tanks buried underground with an estimated 25% leaking. Many industrial chemical tanks also leak and pollute ground water.

Twenty-five to thirty million acres of lawns in the US are fertilized each year. These urban landscapers use two and one-half times more pesticides per acre than do farmers, and the run-off goes into underground water sources. About 20% of all public ground water supplies contain pesticides. Agricultural runoff containing not only pesticides, but fertilizers and animal manure can contaminate water collectors.

In an effort to remove these pollutants, city water suppliers employ elaborate filtration systems. They also add substances such as chlorine, to kill bacteria, and fluoride, to "help" our health. Unfortunately most treatment plants are under funded and therefore water purity is compromised.

Most pollutants in city water can be eliminated in the home, by use of reverse-osmosis systems or distillers. Reverse-osmosis removes lead, copper, nitrates, radium, sodium, and certain pesticides, fungicides and VOC's (volatile organic compounds) and 98% of all contaminants. Distilled water can eliminate bacteria, fluoride, sodium, nitrates, heavy metals and most dissolved solids. They are the only removal methods for toxic gases such as chloroform.

CHLORINE TOXICITY

Chlorine has been praised as the answer to combatting biological pollutants in drinking water and swimming pools. If you were to look at labels concerning chlorine they identify it as a poison with all the necessary precautions mentioned. If a poison is truly effective against unwanted micro-organisms, what can it be doing to the cells inside our bodies and our pets.

Studies show that the cancer risk from chlorine used to treat water could be greater than 1 in 10,000. Chlorine, used to sterilize our water reacts with other organic (carbon-based) materials and produces hundreds of chemical byproducts, several of which cause cancer in animals. These THM's (Trihalomethanes) consist of hundreds of deadly members, among them carbon-tetrachloride, bis-chloroethane and chloroform, all known carcinogens. They are turning up in most cities water supplies.

A U.S. Public Health Service study associated chlorine water ingestion by humans with premature and low birth weight, and increased the risk of bladder and rectal cancer. These studies were conducted with Total Trihalomethanes (chlorine byproducts) of 80 parts per billion. The federal maximum is 100 ppb.

Chlorine can also interact with radioactive substances in water. Carol Keough quotes, in "Water Fit to Drink", "Dr. Carl J. Johnson MD, states that chlorination acts on plutonium, changing it into a more soluble form that is readily absorbed by the intestinal tract, resulting in concentrations in the bone and liver of animals 1,570 times greater than concentrations prior to chlorination."

Jawbone cancer in dogs has been on the increase. Veterinarians are at a loss to find a cause. Maybe a study of those cases would reveal that the water the animals drink is chlorinated. Take precautions to keep your pet from being a statistic and give them filtered water.

The best way to determine if your water source contains chlorine is to use a do-it-yourself test kit that will let you know the presence of chlorine as well as nitrate/nitrites, iron, acidity and hardness. Water filters containing activated carbon have proven effective at removing chlorine, and also gases like chloroform and hydrocarbon organic based chemicals including pesticides, PCB's and the chlorine by-products trihalomethanes. Activated carbon filters can be placed on supply water pipes in the home at the point of use (next to the faucet). These carbon filters have to be monitored, as the absorptive capacity of the carbon eventually is depleted and therefore must be replaced periodically. Most filters last at least six months depending on the level of contamination, and they are not expensive to replace.

Ozone has been used for water treatment since the 18th century. It is one of the best germicides available having the ability to destroy pathogenic organisms such as cysts, virus, amoebae and spores all of which are resistant to chlorine. Europe has been using ozone to treat city water for years and even the city of Los Angeles has used it in its Olympic swimming pool. Many more U.S. cities are now turning to ozone purification and eliminating the hazards associated with chlorination.

Ozone, unlike chlorine, does not produce chlorine by-products, is not corrosive and does not irritate the eyes. Ozone is used for water purification in primarily industrial, commercial and community water applications. Other than being available for water treatment in swimming pools, it is rarely used for home water systems.

LEAD POISONING FROM WATER

Most cases of lead poisoning are identified in dogs who are suspected of chewing lead painted wood. Unfortunately, animals can exhibit symptoms of lead poisoning even if there is no lead paint to be found. Because of this, veterinarians may not be identifying the culprit properly. If your animal is getting lead poisoned from drinking water, you won't know it unless you test your water. If those results come back positive and you notice your pet with odd symptoms, bring this to the attention of your vet so he can perform a lead test on your animal.

Symptoms can include gastric upset, neurological symptoms, anorexia, restlessness, kidney disorders and in dogs, distemper like behavior. EPA reports that 22% of large U.S. water systems exceed the lead action level, mostly in the Northwest, Midwest and Northeast. If you live in these areas especially, use a lead-in-water test kit to determine the presence of this hazard.

Indoor plumbing in the past consisted of lead pipes. When lead began turning up in drinking water, these pipes were replaced by copper. Unfortunately it wasn't until recently that lead solder was also banned, therefore many home copper plumbing systems can still leach lead into the water. Even with a home system that is "pure", you still may be receiving contamination if you are on city water and their piping from sources is made out of lead.

Faucets, especially those that have bronze or brass fittings, can contain lead and as yet there is no regulation banning these. The law forbids leaching of more than half a microgram of lead into every liter of water. Of twenty faucet brands tested by the University of North Carolina, nineteen leached more lead than the law allows. Manufacturers claim they give the consumer plenty of warning and that they meet all state and federal regulations. It would still be prudent to run the water for several minutes prior to taking the first drink of the day, just to help flush any lead out.

Pipes servicing public water systems can produce unhealthy levels of lead in the water. Old service pipes and newer pipes with lead solder contribute to the contamination. The EPA states that as many as thirty million people served by 819 large and medium- sized public water systems could be drinking water with high lead levels. Water systems are required to test for lead in houses served by lead service lines and notify these customers of the hazard. Many do not adequately monitor these systems nor inform their users. The only solution in this case is to use point-of-use or whole house filtration to remove the lead.

Proper lead removal systems for water are reverse-osmosis, distillation, solid block & precoat adsorption filters, and special filters for heavy metal reduction. If Granulated Activated Carbon filters are used by themselves, they do not remove lead. This type of filter media is used by many inexpensive commercial point-of-use filters, and If you are considering purchasing a filter system, specify that you need guarantees that their system will remove lead.

FLUORIDE

Fluoride is added to toothpaste and water as a preventative against dental decay. Americans consume more fluoride than any other group in the world. It was originally introduced because as a byproduct of the manufacture of aluminum, it was discovered that it could be marketed as a reinforcement for dental enamel. Actually, fluoride is a known poison. It has been used as a pesticide and in concentrated form, as a rat poison (which also causes the death of scores of innocent animals). One-tenth of an ounce can cause death in humans. It was banned in many European countries and Australia some time ago.

At 1 part per million it helps prevent tooth decay, and at 2 parts per million, dental fluorosis (staining of the teeth) can occur. At 4 parts per million, fluoride can have an effect on humans whereby they can develop a crippling bone disorder.   The Physicians Desk Reference (for humans) states that fluoride can have the following adverse effects: Eczema, gastric distress, Mongolism, mottling of the teeth and headaches. It has also been reported to exacerbate kidney disease, hypoglycemia, hormonal imbalance, birth defects and even cancer. Dr. Dean Burk, former head chemist of the National Cancer Institute reported to Congress in 1975 that fluoride was linked to over 10,000 cancer deaths in the U.S. each year. Fluoride is thought to change the genetic structure of cells and chromosomes. If humans can develop illness from fluoride, think of what it can cause in our smaller animal family members.

People brush their teeth with fluoride toothpaste, drink water with fluoride added and are treated with fluoride at the dentist. Pets normally only get fluoride in water, unless you brush their teeth, but danger exists when fluoride limits exceed 1 ppm in drinking water (fluoride toothpaste can sometimes have up to 1,000 ppm.).This can have a greater effect on pets who are smaller and ingest more fluoride concentrations per body weight. If your pet develops bone problems, and you have fluoride added to your water (usually city water), advise your veterinarian of your concern about this poison.

The EPA has a limit of 4 parts per million for fluoride in drinking water. The National Academy of Sciences reviewed, studied and determined that this limit should be an "interim" standard until more research is done. EPA requested a review of these standards after an animal study found an elevated rate of bone tumors in male rats exposed to doses of 100 ppm. of fluoride. The EPA panel indicated that dental fluorosis (staining of the teeth) is the only condition likely to arise from consuming excess fluoride in drinking water. If you don't want to wait until the government determines if fluoride is absolutely safe at these limits, you can treat your drinking water by installing a reverse-osmosis filtration system to eliminate extra fluoride from being ingested.

WELL WATER

It is well known that many substances can be inert until they are mixed with others, quite possibly producing extreme reactions and totally new substances. Nitrates from agricultural run-off and septic tank leakage can enter our wells. In farm country, herbicides are used for weed control on a pre-determined schedule, regardless of need and the number of pounds of herbicides needed per acre is growing every year.

When we drink this substance it can be transformed inside the mouth into compounds called nitrosamines. In studies with rats, these have caused cancer. Well water normally doesn't contain chlorine or fluoride, but there are no guarantees that other contaminants are not seeping into your water source. Sulfur, normally found in shallow wells, is not necessarily harmful, but it's foul odor can deter pets from drinking the water thereby promoting dehydration.

The best way to verify contamination levels in well water is have a test performed. If you are worried about nitrates-nitrites you can do a home test with an over the counter kit. If you would like to know all the pollutants in your water then hire a professional to perform a complete test. It is not practical to do this on a monthly basis, and since pollutants may come and go, the best assurance for safe water is whole house or point-of-use filtration. Before deciding on which type of filter is necessary, review your water test results with a water treatment expert.

BOTTLED WATER

The University of Tennessee Agricultural Extension Service discovered that bottled water is not necessarily safer than tap water. Bottled water is checked by the Food and Drug Administration, not the EPA. The FDA tests bottled water only when a consumer complains, and has found that 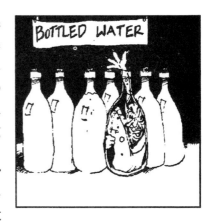 many of the manufacturers do not comply with US drinking standards.

The Food and Drug Administration has set standards for bottled water that allow certain levels of 35 inorganic and synthetic organic chemicals, 11 synthetic volatile organic chemicals, 14 pesticides and PCBs. There are no limits for certain pesticides or asbestos. Any of these contaminants could be found in bottled water therefore most bottled water manufacturers are now running their source through reverse-osmosis units before bottling to remove the contamination. Unless spring water is routinely tested or run through a purifier, it also can contain contaminants.

These products can be considered safe unless they have been stored for a period of time in a warm warehouse where they could breed bacteria. It is essential that as a consumer, you don't assume that bottled water is free from contamination. Contact the manufacturer and request a water test result report to be sure.

MINERAL DEFICIENT WATER

Reverse-osmosis and distillation will take nearly 100% of the dissolved solids out of water, including minerals which are necessary for your pet's health. This water has been called "dead" because it lacks the life force nature puts in. Unfortunately we have a choice either to have water with minerals and toxic chemicals, or eliminate all dissolved solids and add back the minerals. Obviously, we don't want the toxic pollutants to be a part of our pet's diet, therefore the second option is the only real choice.

Minerals and electrolytes are really the spark of life. Electrolytes are the basis of good health and are used in the maintenance and repair of all tissue, utilization of amino acids and are the basis of every physical and neurological function. They maintain "osmotic equilibrium", the internal water balance that enables mucus and nerves to contract and expand and wounds to heal.

Electrolytes are also essential for growth and development of the bones and organs. Neither muscles nor nerves function properly, unless they are bathed in tissue fluids which contain mineral salts. Electrolytes also act to potentiate and increase absorption of vitamins, macro minerals and proteins (amino acids) from food and natural supplements such as kelp, garlic, yeast, cod liver oil and wheat germ oil.

It's absolutely necessary to supplement your pet's diet with minerals and electrolytes, either by adding it to your purified water or their food.

COMMON WATER CONTAMINANTS
& ASSOCIATED HEALTH EFFECTS

Microbiologicals	Digestive disorders, fever
Arsenic	Tumors, nervous system
Barium	Nervous & Circulatory Systems
Cadmium	Kidney, Bronchitis, Anemia
Copper	Stomach, Intestines
Cyanide	Thyroid, Nervous System
Fluoride	Fluorosis
Lead	Nervous system, Kidney
Pesticides	Nervous system, Kidneys, Liver Cancer, Heart
Organic chemicals	Kidneys, Liver, Lungs, Cancer Nervous System

BUILDING & DECORATING
HAZARDS

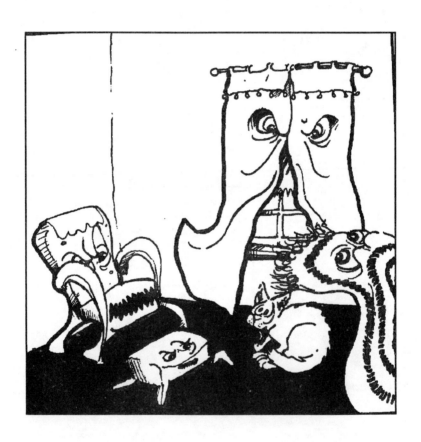

This chapter is written as food for thought. Many manufacturers will dispute the information presented, after all, they have a vested interest in doing so. Grandma used to say, "everything is safe in moderation". Unfortunately we do not breathe indoor air in moderation and most of it is toxic. Therefore it is not safe for pets or humans. Even moderate amounts of chemical inhalation can cause lifetime sickness in certain people.

It has only been in recent years that indoor environmental building and decorating materials have been considered hazardous. Carpets, plastics and volatile organic compounds in paint, have been criticized for outgassing dangerous fumes. Many symptoms attributed to these toxins, can appear in your pets before they appear in you. As cats and dogs are closer to the source for longer periods of time, they can breathe in higher concentrations of chemicals for their given body weight.

Studies on animals have confirmed human sickness from indoor contaminants is real. Sensitive people, asthmatics, etc., react more violently to chemical fumes, but any "sick building" inhabitant, including animals, can develop mild symptoms. Medical professionals are normally not schooled in the identification of these airborne toxins, therefore they may mis-diagnose the problem and treat patients without success.

Manufacturers are either recognizing the hazards of their product ingredients or complying with new state laws, but either way they are beginning to create safer building and decorating materials. Low Volatile Organic Compound (VOC) paint has recently appeared on the commercial market, in addition to already established "natural" paints.

Natural wool, jute and sisal carpets have always been available, but it has only been in the last few years that they have become price competitive. Synthetic carpet manufacturers have established a limit for toxic emissions and may indicate safer carpets on the labels. The plastics industry continues to develop innovative ways to get their toxic products into our homes. If you worry about the effect of fumes outgassing from plastic based furniture, flooring, storage containers, etc. investigate more natural alternatives. Formaldehyde is one of the largest culprits for creating interior gas chambers. Most of our "fake wood" furniture uses formaldehyde glue. Drapes, sofas, bedding, carpets and cabinets contain this chemical. Outgassing diminishes as time goes by, but by then your pet, and you, can already have been affected. The cotton industry has flourished lately, due to desire for chemical free clothing and bedding.

There is light at the end of the tunnel and it starts with education. As building inhabitants learn more about these toxins the better equipped they will be to choose alternative products. Since pets can't read, it is up to their owners to protect them. Poisoning your pet slowly from indoor air contamination is as malicious as giving them a strychnine meatball.

SYMPTOMS FROM
BUILDING MATERIALS

COUGH

NAUSEA

NERVOUSNESS

DEPRESSION

BREATHING PROBLEMS

SKIN RASH

CANCER

ANXIETY

IRRITABILITY

SYNTHETIC CARPETS

SYNTHETIC CARPET INGREDIENTS
*Excerpted from Hendricksen Naturlich flooring brochure

Ethylbenzene	1-ethyl-3-methylbenzene
Formaldehyde	Hexadecanol
Mithacrylic acid	Hexamethylene triamine
Methyl methacrylate	10H-indene
Tetrachloroethylene	1-methylnaphtalene
Toluene	2-methylnaphtalene
Xylenes	5-methyltridecane
4-phenylcyclohexene	Octadecenyl amine
Acetonitrile	Oxarium
Azulene	1-phenylcyclopentanol
Benzene	2-propylheptanol
Biphenyl	Ptalic esters
2-butyloctanol-1	Styrene
1,3,5 cycloheptatriene	1,2,3-trimethylbenzene
Diphenyl ether	Tetradecene
Dodecane	Undecane

Mr. and Mrs. Spider took their kids on a journey inside a fancy house every Sunday. There were no big problems except the occasional scurrying to avoid 'big foot' walking across the floor, until one day when the spiders, upon entering the house, smelled something very dangerous. Mr. 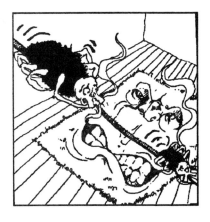 Spider knew that if they continued on their normal path they would become very sick. They avoided the new carpet in the living room, choosing to walk around on the hardwood floor. They still did not like the smell and felt it would be better to avoid this house in the future. Subsequently, the owners began to get sick and thought it might be the carpet so they removed it. Somehow Mr. and Mrs. Spider found out and came back to the house, retracing their original steps over the old wood floor. This is a true story from two different families who found that their new carpet had made them sick. Maybe we should pay more attention to these prehistoric creatures.

Even in the Environmental Protection Agency, problems from new carpet arose. In 1987 they installed 27,000 yards of carpet in one of their office complexes. Eighteen months later, after scores of complaints and reported illness from the workers, the carpet was removed. Although they said they were unable to establish scientific evidence linking the sickness with the carpet, their action (removing the carpet) spoke for itself.

4-PC is a glue which has been used in most synthetic carpets, to affix the backing to the carpet. This glue has proven to be highly toxic. Fortunately, many manufacturers are currently eliminating the use of 4-PC. Read the label on the carpet to be sure. Other chemicals such as formaldehyde, toluene, xylene, tetrachloroethylene, styrene, ethylbenzene, phtalic esters and many more are found in carpets. Would you give these chemicals to your pet in their water dish? If not, why are you exposing them to fumes coming from the flooring?

Humans develop the following symptoms from synthetic carpet fumes: burning eyes, chills, sore throat, cough, nausea, dizziness, nervousness and depression. If your pets could talk, they may tell you they have the same symptoms. Since it is difficult to determine if your cat or dog has burning eyes or depression, you may have to resort to watching their behavior, especially if you have recently had a new synthetic carpet installed. A safer alternative both for your pets and your family is to install non-toxic wool, jute or sisal carpets or to choose hardwood floors instead.

If it is impossible for you to remove your existing new carpet, consider purchasing an air treatment device which can effectively eliminate the fumes. You can also apply non-toxic sprays which lock in the toxins and reduce their emissions.

FORMALDEHYDE

Formaldehyde has been proven to cause cancer in animals. People have been affected by formaldehyde fumes indicated by the following symptoms: watery eyes, sore throat, nausea, skin rash, cough, tiredness, excessive thirst, nosebleeds, and difficulty breathing.

Should your pet exhibit any of these symptoms, consider formaldehyde poisoning if you have recently redecorated. Outgassing fumes are at their strongest when building or decorating materials are new. High indoor temperatures and humidity levels can increase the release of these gases.

This toxin is found in many products including flue, adhesive, paint preservatives, pressed wood products, fabric finishes, paneling and even unvented fuel-burning appliances. Your cat or dog can be affected by formaldehyde fumes if you keep them in a tightly closed 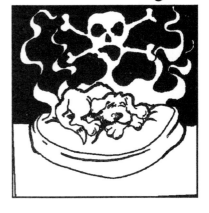 house without proper air circulation and ventilation.

Fumes from new particleboard furniture, carpets, and paneling can add to indoor air pollution. Many sofa, draperies or bedding materials have fabric finishes such as permanent press and stain resistant coatings. These can be formaldehyde-based and any pet sleeping on these surfaces can become affected. Cats and dogs sleep longer and more often than you do. If their bed or sleeping place (on your bed) has chemicals in the fabric, they will be breathing them for a greater period of time. Pets have much more opportunity to become contaminated, especially if they spend most of their time indoors.

There are home test kits available to determine levels of formaldehyde in your house, but they may be unreliable. If you suspect a problem you should call a professional lab to perform the proper evaluation; alternatives to toxic products are available. Solid wood furniture is still made. Natural cotton bedding and fabric coverings are a suitable solution, as are natural carpets or hardwood flooring. A simple immediate solution would be to purchase an air treatment device to remove these noxious fumes.

PAINT

No one considered paint a bad substance until it was discovered that lead could cause illness, especially in children. Lead paint was outlawed and we thought we were safe until more research found another culprit, volatile organic compounds (VOC). These toxins can contribute to smog and ozone pollution as well affecting the health of pets and their owners.

VOCs are used commonly as ingredients in paint, varnish, stain, strippers and also in all-purpose cleaners, degreasing and hobby products, moth repellents and air fresheners. Common side effects of breathing these toxic fumes are respiratory irritation, kidney problems, asthma, wheezing and croup. Animals can have other symptoms which are difficult to diagnose such as visual disorders, depression and memory impairment. Ingredients like methylene chloride, benzene and perchloroethylene have proven to cause cancer in animals. The Environmental Protection Agency produced a study that showed that many of these organic pollutants have five times the concentration inside our buildings than outside.

The obvious solution to protecting our pets from inadvertent poisoning from VOCs is to eliminate the usage of these products. Many substitutes are available in the form of low VOC paint and varnish, and natural air fresheners found in health food stores.

Use cedar shavings instead of mothballs, baking soda or vinegar and salt as all purpose cleaners. As repeated throughout this chapter, it is important to remove these gases from your interior through a proper air purification device.

VOCs can also be found in water. As these compounds evaporate rapidly during normal household activities such as dish washing, doing the laundry, flushing the toilet and taking a shower, proper precautions should be taken. A carbon adsorption type of point-of-use water filter can be installed in your home and remove VOCs as long as the filter is maintained and changed properly. Remember, you not only may jeopardize your pets' health through the water you give them, but by your use of toxic products that contaminate the air they breathe.

SUNLIGHT INDOORS

Another indoor pollutant, so to speak, can cause Seasonal Affective Disorder (SAD). Light pollution is not feared as causing cancer or physical sickness, but it can trigger extreme mood swings and depression in humans during winter months. Animals confined to ordinarily lit 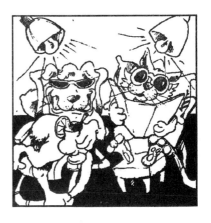 houses or kennels do not have the advantage of copious amounts of sunlight which stimulates essential biological functions.

During winter months, your pets may become lethargic, increase their appetite and put on weight. This could be due to the lack of full spectrum light found naturally in sunlight. If your pet is outside a good bit of time, they may not experience this disorder, but animals confined to a mostly interior lighting environment are susceptible.

Zoos have discovered that birds, fish and other animals have had their health improved when simulated sunlight was introduced. Conventional lighting emits an overabundance of yellow light which can promote anxiety, depression, fatigue and irritability. Light affects menstrual regularity and fertility in animals due to bright light causing the irregular release of the hormone, melatonin.

The simple solution is to install full spectrum light bulbs, commonly known as plant grow lights. These bulbs mimic daylight and should cause an improvement in your pets spirits. Chicken farmers have discovered that when they installed full spectrum lights, the birds acted less aggressively. The cholesterol content of their eggs was also reduced and their productive life lengthened. Full spectrum lights are listed in the resource directory chapter in this book.

SOLUTIONS

The simplest solution is to go back to nature and live without these toxic materials. Unfortunately that is impractical, and even if you became a purist, toxins would filter in from outside. We do recommend substituting toxic cleaners and pesticides for non-toxic methods, but interior decorating materials must be compromised. It is almost impossible to find current building products that are chemical free. Therefore, you must attack them from within your home.

Non-toxic carpets still can harbor mold which may cause skin and respiratory irritations in your pets. Non-toxic cleaners and paints will still be hazardous if swallowed by your dog or cat. People who smoke can cause illness through secondary cigarette smoke and the butts in the ashtray are toxic to birds who may find them attractive as food or playthings. Fumes from your furnace can cause problems and you may have to compromise by buying permanent press drapes or sofas. Therefore you should budget for purchasing an air treatment device.

Many air treatment units are effective at removing noxious gasses, zapping pollutants out of the air, and keeping mold at bay. One type uses natural ozone (extra oxygen molecule) combined with a negative ionizer and are effective at reducing allergies in kennels and aviaries and putting a smile on your pet's face. The ozone attaches to airborne particles and converts them to harmless compounds which fall to the floor or dissipate. The negative ions promote a sense of well-being in the animals, such as one finds after a thunderstorm has cleared the air. Birds seem to stop picking their feathers and dogs have even been found to stop scratching because of reduction by the air purification device, of allergic contamination in the air.

Electrostatic units use negative and positive ions to attract contaminants to the air cleaner unit, where they are caught in a removable filter. Still others use sophisticated HEPA (high efficiency particulate arrestor) and carbon filters to clean gas and particulate from the air. Information on specific air treatment devices are given in the Resource Directory section of this book. You should analyze your specific needs and choose a unit that is specific to that application.

Air circulation is important in your home and grandma was right when she always opened the windows. Today, it costs too much to heat our homes, therefore we don't want to open windows and our homes remain stuffy toxic gas chambers. If you are adamant about keeping your dwelling shut tight, then consider installing a heat recovery ventilation system or air circulation fan system to exchange the air many times every hour. Clean air is essential to our pets' health. If they develop illness because of your "sick building" syndrome, the rest of your family will surely follow.

KEEPING PETS HEALTHY

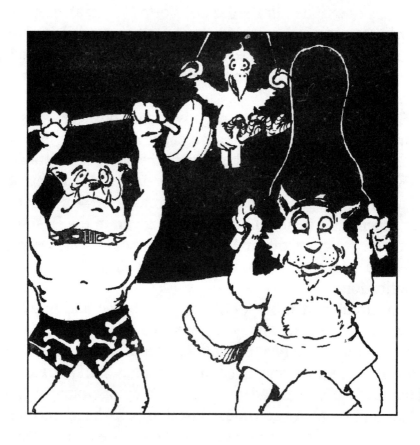

There are many solutions to keeping your pet healthy. As in all disease, it is important to diagnose the cause before recommending treatment. Once that cause is determined, solutions can be implemented which will prevent reinfection. The best defense against most toxins is to keep your pet's immune system at its peak. Weakness in this area can be attributed to poor diet, lack of exercise, depletion of trace minerals and proper enzymes.

DIET

Information is being written on the hazards of commercial pet foods, being about as good for your animal as processed and fast foods are for humans. Many pet foods contain low quality ingredients rejected for human consumption and are highly processed with questionable chemical 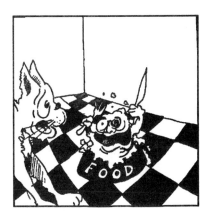 additives. Vitamins and minerals are deficient or depleted in processing.

Advertising claims of 'complete and balanced' are based on uncertain minimum nutritional requirements designed merely for adequate health, not optimum health. No wonder so many pets become prematurely sick. Wise owners supplement their animals diet, but beware: pet supplements can be made with low quality ingredients and potentially allergenic substances for sensitive animals, such as brewers yeast, milk, wheat, artificial flavors and dyes. These substances can cause scratching, skin problems and diarrhea, therefore read labels and avoid products with these ingredients.

Birds eat to balance their energy needs. Some veterinarians say that because the minimum nutrient requirements for parrots are not known, feed companies cannot claim that they have a complete diet. The proof is how healthy the bird looks and acts. Sickly birds show signs of feather stress bars, poor pigmentation, thinness, or obesity and weak bones. High fat diets can cause wet and smelly droppings. They usually have been fed seed with minimum levels of essential fatty acids and amino acids necessary for maintenance of energy levels. Microbial contamination of seed is another problem area, usually handled through avoidance of animal byproducts, fish, or eggs which can contain the organisms. Since microbial contamination can harm baby birds (when their immune system is poorly developed), it is wise to confront your seed supplier and ask if they test for bacteria counts. Information on companion bird diets can be obtained through Hagen Avicultural Research Institute, P.O. Box 490, Riguad, Quebec Canada J0P 1P0.

Wild birds must also be fed complete diets using seed continuing no additives or fillers. We may think we are being helpful to wild birds by feeding through the winter, but we usually stop when the first spring flower arrives. This is a particularly crucial time for birds as their normal stores of winter seed are gone and plants are not producing replacements yet. Please continue to feed your wild birds in the spring and also in the summer, when you could make their life easier when they are preoccupied with finding enough feed for their young.

Many pet owners feed pets "people food". Be discriminating in what kind of table scraps you offer your pets. Liver, if more than 10% of a cat's diet (too much vitamin A), can lead to distorted bones, gingivitis, tooth problems and stiff joints. Beware also of giving raw fish and raw eggs to your cat as they contains an enzyme, thiaminase which inactivates Vitamin B1. If you feed your pet only one type of food (all beef, all chicken, etc.) you may need to supplement their diet with vitamins.

Vegetarians sometimes believe they must make their animals non-meat eaters as well. Most animals do not thrive on vegetarian diets. Cats especially need taurine, an amino-acid like substance found in meat and fish. Without this substance, the cat may develop degeneration of the heart muscle and possibly go blind. Dogs tolerate all vegetable diets better as they are able to synthesize sufficient quantities of taurine. Balanced diets are best, although I would avoid meat and fish contaminated with pesticides, hormones and heavy metals.

Green foods are so important to your pet's diet because of the beneficial enzymes added and life giving force. For example, chlorophyll is an internal antiseptic, a cell stimulator, red blood builder and rejuvenator. It relieves respiratory troubles and discomforts in the sinus and lungs and is beneficial to blood and heart conditions. The best source of chlorophyll is alfalfa along with barley grass, wheatgrass, blue-green algae, and spirulina. Barley grass contains a compound, Tocopherol Acid Succinate which has the potential of preventing the body's immune system from breaking down while fighting off disease that cripples the body's natural system of defense. Also good for the immune system are parsley, nutritional yeast and Cod liver oil (vitamin A and D). Some herbal supplements which will support the immune system are garlic (digestion), nettles (skin), burdock (digestive cleanser), hawthorn (heart), buchu (bladder), oats (nervous system), and celery seed (muscles and joints). Products containing any of these nutrients are valuable additives to your pets' diet and will ultimately enhance their health.

If you are interested in learning which diet is nutritionally correct for your pet, we suggest contacting a veterinarian. Names of those that specialize in holistic approaches to diet can be obtained from The American Holistic Veterinary Medical Association, 2214 Old Emmorton Rd., Bel Air, MD 21014 (410)-569-0795.

EXERCISE

Exercise is as important to your pet as it is to you. Couch potato animals run similar risk of heart ailments as do humans, especially if they have been fed a high fat diet. People rarely exercise their indoor pets and are usually overfeeding them. Animals, especially dogs, will beg for 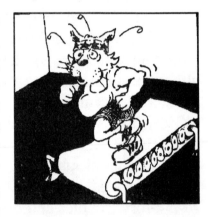 food and if their demands are constantly met, they can be plagued with obesity. Putting an animal on a diet may seem cruel when those pitiful eyes watch you eat your succulent dinner, but it may be necessary. A word of caution: before implementing any dietary regime, contact your veterinarian for advice.

Be conscious of your pets athletic ability. Dogs in tip top shape may be able to jog the seven miles with you, but if they are not used to exercise, permanent damage could follow. Animals, like humans, have to build up to exercise, therefore be conscious of their limits. Even though dogs want to please and will try to keep up with you when bicycling or running, don't let them unless you know they're fit.

MINERALS

Animals and humans today have a marked disadvantage over living creatures from the past. We are lacking proper amounts of trace minerals. During the glacier age, mineral rich soil was deposited over the planet. Erosion and chemical farming methods have caused depletion of trace 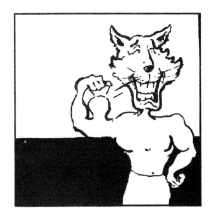 minerals from topsoil, and from the plants grown in this soil. Polluted water is filtered, most times eliminating what minerals are left in it. When trace minerals are deficient in our food and water, the body's defense systems cannot function properly, allowing toxins to build up and increase susceptibility to infection. Animals lacking proper amounts of copper, iron, selenium , etc. have been found to be associated with an increased risk of cancer. Mineral deficient pets exposed to the poisons we have spoken about in this book are much more likely to develop disease.

Sick animals are usually given drugs and vitamins. Vitamins are fortifiers. They control the body's appropriation of minerals, and in the absence of minerals they have no function to perform and therefore are useless. Putting minerals back in your pet's diet is essential.

Crystalloid minerals were administered to race horses in upstate New York. (Crystalloid means that minerals bypass the digestive process and are absorbed directly into cell walls, strengthening the immune system.) A marked improvement was seen in the animals' behavior. The horses were much more alert, less nervous and jumpy.

Their coats improved, and one horse with a two year old bare patch of skin from a prior injury began to grow back his hair. Muscle soreness and stiffness disappeared, and their racing ability improved.

Proteins are not well assimilated if trace minerals are deficient. This is important since most of our pet foods are meat-based. You may be feeding your dog but still starving him nutritionally if he is unable to process the food. Properly balanced minerals with electrolytes would be a wise investment to keep your pet's immune system working correctly. Supplementing your pet's diet with individual minerals may not be the best way of attacking this problem as you may not be administering the required dose for his needs or you may be upsetting his mineral balance. To your pet's diet add a mineral supplement that contains all the needed minerals in the proper amounts.

ENZYMES

Enzymes are catalysts for many biological functions. Without them life would not exist, for they are the driving force behind all life processes. They are responsible for keeping your internal systems working, and a lack of sufficient quantities of enzymes promotes degenerative disease. Only raw or uncooked foods contain enzymes and since almost all pet food is processed with heat, or cooked, the enzymes are destroyed. Every animal is born with an integral supply of enzymes. Unfortunately, as generations go by and less enzymes are taken into the body, those stores are used up.

Dr. Edward Howell, as early as 1920, discovered this association between enzyme intake and health. He theorized that normally, food enzymes are used for the digestion of that food. If they are not present, then the body stores of enzymes must be diverted for digestion, leaving fewer enzymes to fight disease and perform essential bodily functions.

Research indicates that most animals, including canines and birds, have distinct organs that allow the food enzymes time to act before initiating the body's own digestive process. This pre-digestion is important to the body's absorption of nutrients. If it is not present, then food may pass through the system without benefit of vitamins and proteins.

A study of Dr. Francis Pottenger's cats revealed that over many generations, degenerative disease presented itself at younger and younger ages, when the animals were fed only cooked or processed food. They had fewer enzymes to give their offspring resulting in minimal reserves of enzymes in the ensuing generations. We have seen this evidenced in the early onset of arthritic conditions. Your pets may live as long, but their quality of life suffers. These animals suffered from kidney, heart, thyroid and gum diseases as well as allergies, infections and a host of other maladies.

Enzymes are normally lost through sickness, pregnancy, stress, extreme weather conditions, urine and feces. Unless you replace these stores, your pet's immune system will be compromised. Please note that this is the same for humans, exhibited by our younger generations developing earlier cases of heart disease, arthritis and susceptibility to allergies. It is necessary to consider supplementing your pet's diet with nutritional enzymes if they depend on canned or dried food.

HERBS

Solutions to disease in pets should be left to the expertise of the veterinarian, but the treatments mentioned in this section may replace drug therapy and should be considered. Veterinarians may already know about herbal "cures", but if not, you may be able to open their eyes.

The following listing of herbs is reprinted in part, from the May-June, 1994 edition of Natural Pet Magazine and is for educational purposes only. It is not provided in order to diagnose, prescribe, or treat any disease, illness, or injured condition of the body in humans or in animals. The authors, publishers, printers, distributors accept no responsibility for such use.

ARTHRITIS/RHEUMATIC CONDITIONS

Alfalfa helps to alkalize the body and is high in chlorophyll and nutrients. It's anti-rheumatic effect is probably due to its high nutritive value. Couchgrass and lavender are also used for patients suffering from rheumatism. A poultice of rosemary leaves or a hot compress of the tea can be

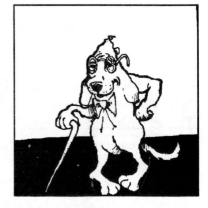

used for arthritic joints. Garlic has been useful in relieving pain from arthritis or dysplasia as well. Use 1/2 to 3 cloves with each meal. An oat straw bath is useful for relief of joint pain. Nettles have an anti-inflammatory action to reduce swelling and pain. Yucca has been used to manage the pain of soft tissue inflammation. Parsley can also be sprinkled into their meal which strengthens, especially the cat's body and gives a good supportive base for chronic cases.

BITES AND CUTS

Almost every owner of an outdoor pet has had to contend with their animal receiving a bite, which becomes an abscess. Echinacea is an anti-bacterial herb that can assist in prevention of infection and stimulate the animal's immune system. Witch Hazel, used topically, has an astringent action that can stop bleeding and reduces inflammation and bruising. Arnica is good for bruises and sprains. Calendula, diluted in lotion form, can be applied to wounds that have closed. It stimulates healing and reduces pain and inflammation. A word of caution not to apply calendula to open wounds as it may assist scabbing over too early and prevent any abscess from draining. Diluted woundwort is used to cleanse wounds or in a compress to cover the sore. Comfrey can also be used as a poultice, especially for deep wounds. Dr. Bach's Five Flower Combination formula, Calming Essence. can be used in cream form to the injured area.

BEE STINGS

Fat lips are common in animals that find amusement in chasing bees. If your animal gets stung, you can apply aloe, either fresh from the plant in your house or in bottled juice form. Lavender and eucalyptus oils can reduce pain and swelling. If it is known that the sting came from a 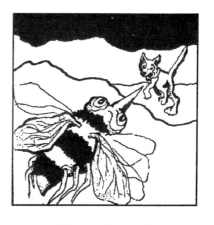 wasp, apply thyme vinegar as an antidote. Regular bee stings can be treated with sodium bicarbonate dissolved in ice water.

CYSTITIS

Animals are frequently found straining to urinate and licking their "privates". This is often a symptom of a urinary tract infection that restricts the urethra and causes a pinching or burning sensation. It can be caused by too much ash in dried pet foods or from a bacteria. Several herbs are successful in treating this condition. Buchu helps dissolve gravel and promote urination as well as treating incontinence. Having astringent and antiseptic qualities, barberry soothes and strengthens the urinary tract. Parsley teas promote the flow of urine, helps remove gravel and can soothe the area irritated in the urinary trace. Mugwort and gravel oak can also be helpful.

DIARRHEA

Capsicum is a natural stimulant for diarrhea and dysentery. If there is gas with simple constipation, try giving some Carboveg (vegetable charcoal). Chamomile is safe for all animals and is an excellent nervine, making it especially useful in treating digestive problems produced by anxiety. Garlic can disinfect the digestive tract and assist in restoration of friendly bacteria. Barberry stimulates the liver and promotes the flow of bile which can return the bowel to normal.

DIGESTION

Caraway seed tea aids digestion as does chamomile, gentian and the yucca plant. Burdock root is alkalizing and soothing to the stomach and intestines. Couchgrass (also known as Doggrass, Twitchgrass and Quickgrass) leaves are much sought after by many kinds of animals as a spring tonic. Dogs and cats eat couch leaves to promote vomiting, or as a laxative. Birds and poultry eat the seeds for treatment of all bladder ailments, gallstones and constipation. The silica content of couchgrass helps to strengthen teeth, beaks and claws. Some herbs such as Dandelion and Fennel are known as Stomachicherbs. They are usually bitter in flavor and are used to help promote and improve digestion and appetite. Slippery Elm (powdered bark) can be made into a syrup and is well known for its help with digestion. Peppermint oil will soothe the stomach lining and reduce the urge to vomit, and reduce gas. Chamomile can also reduce gas and soothe the digestive system. Black walnut expels internal parasites and tapeworms. For hairballs (cats) use a combination of either psyllium, licorice root and hibiscus flowers or aloe vera juice with liquid chlorophyll.

MUSCLE SPASMS

Cayenne, Fennel, Lavender and Sage are known to help with muscle spasms. Oats are a tonic, particularly for animals that exhibit twitching, paralysis or tremors. For muscle pain, you can apply rosemary. Use 1 teaspoon of the herb in a cup of boiling water. Apply when cool. Add 1 to 2 drops of hazelnut or lavender oil and work into the affected area.

RESPIRATORY

Comfrey can be used as an expectorant to remove mucus from the intestinal tract. Garlic has great anti-viral properties and is best known for its effectiveness in treating lung ailments. Anise is helpful in removing excess mucus. The oils in garlic are excreted through the respiratory tract and are good for bronchitis. Coltsfoot is an anti-spasmodic and expectorant with anti-inflammatory properties due to its zinc content, and is useful in treating cases of bronchitis and cough. White horehound combines well with coltsfoot for bronchitis as it dilates the airways and helps to loosen mucous. Schlsandra is used in blends for coughing, wheezing or asthma.

SKIN CONDITIONS
Burdock root is cooked like a carrot and used as a blood purifier. Calendula can be used topically. Dry, itchy skin is an indication of many problems and animals suffering from this problem usually have bladder inflammation and pain. Make an infusion of sarsaparilla rootstock in one cup of near boiling water, strain and give proportionally from 2 tsp. for a small animal up to 6 tablespoons to a giant dog, three times daily.

FLOWER AND PLANT REMEDIES
The Yucca plant has been gaining a lot of attention in pet food manufacturing circles because of its stool deodorizer properties, but it has been therapeutically used of centuries. It is an excellent anti-inflammatory and proven to be a very safe and effective substitute for steroid-based medications. It is effective in reducing the itch response in allergic animals and if used topically, to support tissue healing and reduced scarring. Flower remedies are especially useful in treating emotional and stress disorders in animals. In the form of liquids or creams, they can be used for any immediate solution that is stressing or traumatizing the animal, and can be used to help stabilize all large and small birds, animals and fish, before, during, and after any traumatic situation, even for car sickness.

Flower remedies also work well for reducing pain, swelling and inflammation of skin disorders, insect bites, burns, bruises and sprains.

IMPATIENS
For uptight, impatient, irritable animals.

MIMULUS

For timid, frightened animals afraid of known things such as water, thunder, riding in cars, etc.

ASPEN

For animals the are fearful of the unknown, their surroundings and circumstances

CHESTNUT BUD

For animals who have difficulty learning lessons during training, to help correct wrong habits and negative repetitive behavior.

OLIVE

For exhaustion resulting from trauma or prolonged sickness.

STAR OF BETHLEHEM

For trauma or grief or for animals that have been injured or abused.

ESSENTIAL FATTY ACIDS

Dr. Michael Gazsi, ND, Oxford, CT, is a strong believer in the importance of essential fatty acids for preventative medicine. The following is text from one of his many lectures on the subject.

"Another often overlooked nutrient that is essential to life is EFA (essential fatty acids). These fats, known as Omega 3 and Omega 6, cannot be made by the body but have to be ingested as food. Commercial pet foods are very poor sources of EFAs. Oils containing EFAs are easily damaged by heat, light and oxygen. The heat used to make sure the food contains no bacteria, and the long exposure of the oils to air and light in storage, cause the remaining EFA's to be damaged to the point where they are no longer beneficial nutrients. In fact, they become "trans fats" which are detrimental to the animals' health by inhibiting the normal oils' function in the body.

It has long been known that essential fatty acid deficiency causes dry flaky skin, increased susceptibility to cutaneous infections and hair loss in dogs. Linoleic acid supplementation can lessen the severity of the condition and can correct the fatty acid imbalance in the skin.

Omega 3 and Omega 6 properly balanced in their unadulterated form, are necessary for:

1. The building blocks of membranes in every cell in the body,

2. Energy metabolism as they are used to make a hormone family called prostaglandins,

3. Cardiovascular health, as well as bowel and immune function,

4. Preventative for cancers, diabetes, arthritis, asthma, all inflammatory tissue conditions, skin conditions, visual function, fertility to name a few.

With these in mind, it would be wise to supplement the animal's diet with EFAs on a daily basis in their food. One source of EFA is in oil form. Cold pressed flax seed oil, fish oils, including cod liver oil, borage oil and evening primrose oil, Sunflower and safflower oil are excellent if bought truly cold pressed in dark containers. Unfortunately most cold pressed oils today are heated at some point to control shelf life.

Flax seed if eaten as a whole grain or ground into a powder, is an excellent alternative to oils. It also is a healthy source of protein (contains 8 amino acids), complex carbohydrates (to regulate protein and fat metabolism), vitamins, minerals and provides roughage (to

94

remove toxins and bile cholesterol via elimination).

CLEAN INDOOR AIR AND IONS

Suspecting that our pets are being poisoned by our indoor air giving them oral antidotes is not enough to prevent the problem from recurring. Toxins remain airborne as long as your house is shut tight, obviously being more of a problem during the heating season or if central air conditioning is installed. Air treatment and air exchange are an important part of the cure.

Animals that live in confined indoor environments are just as susceptible to airborne aggravants as are humans. They can develop allergies and respiratory conditions, sometimes at a higher rate because they are closer to the floor where much of the dust accumulates.

Forced air systems blow dust and toxins around. They may cause additional illness because of bacteria that can live in the ductwork. If you have one of these systems in your house, please have the ducts cleaned each year before the heating or air conditioning season begins. Hot water and electric baseboard heating is much cleaner, but still can move the air around (hot air rises) and even fry the dust that lands on the hot pipes, releasing toxins into the air.

Overhead electric radiant panels are known as allergy-free heat. Similar to the effect you would get if you stood in the sun, these solid-state panels warm objects therefore keeping the heat down low where you need it. Animals don't mind sleeping on the floor which is usually kept warm. Since these panels are face mounted to the ceiling, there is no chance for dust to burn on them and because air circulation is kept to a minimum, less dust is airborne for pets to breathe.

Air treatment is an absolute must for well insulated houses. Unless you have furnished your home with natural products, toxic fumes from carpets, stuffed furniture, new drapes or paint will be present. If these airborne hazards are not removed, you and your pets may develop health symptoms. There are many different types of air filtration devices which remove a variety of pollutants. HEPA, carbon and electrostatic filters capture most particles and many gases that pass through them depending on the density of the filter and the size of the dust. Another type of air treatment device is a negative ion generator which zaps dust particles and the toxic gas attached to them. If ion generation is combined with oxidation, the ozone produced in combination with the ions attach themselves to the pollutant and neutralize it. The ozone breaks down these polluted molecules, such as hydrocarbons, into water vapor and carbon dioxide, rendering them harmless. These units have been successfully used in kennels to reduce the level of infection transmission.

Ions are an important part of the well-being of animals and people. Before a thunderstorm, animals exhibit nervous and jittery behavior and upon its passage, seem to calm down. This is due to the fact that before the storm there is a high concentration of positive ions in the air caused by friction, the atmosphere, dust and pollution. Once the storm cleans the air through electrical discharge, negative ions are produced and a sense of calm prevails. Heavy doses of positive ions tend to overstimulate animals. If prolonged periods of positive ions are present, animals can develop behavioral changes and breathing difficulties.

Thousands of experiments have been performed in the last seventy years on the effects of positive and negative ions, which are presumed to be absorbed through the lungs and effect metabolic and glandular systems. The full moon causes a proliferation of positive ions in the air, during which time animals may become anxious, restless and more vocal. Negative ions are reported to create the opposite effect and allow the body to function better. Europeans have long known about the effects of positive ions through their "Witches Winds". Blowing down from mountains at certain periods in the seasons, these winds caused an increase in traffic accidents and hospital patient deaths, more suicides and more domestic violence.

Our current chemically dependent building product manufacturing industry is allowing an ion upset in our homes similar to the effect of the "Witches Winds". Permanent press and synthetic fabrics can cause the common "static cling" which is positive ions interacting with the negative ground. Animals exhibit this same phenomena when their fur becomes "electrified" during dry winter indoor atmospheres. Adding moisture through humidification can help alleviate this problem.

Buildings with forced air systems create harmful positive ions because of metal pipes, blowers, filters and ducting stripping the air of negative ions before it reaches its destination. This is especially evident in skyscrapers. The American Broadcasting Company recognizes behavioral changes in employees from positive ionization and is equipping its New York headquarters with ion control. Philco and Emerson Electric already have ion-control air conditioning systems on the market with other manufacturers following.

Ions have been the object of many medical studies the results of which indicated that patients showed signs of improved recovery, less pain, better moods and less reaction to allergens when negative ions were present. Negative Ions also have a biological effect on bacteria and, in killing these germs, clean the air.

Installing a negative ionizer in conjunction with an air cleaner can reduce or eliminate these effects and keep pets calmer and healthier. Aviaries report that air treatment devices with negative ion generators have kept birds from picking their feathers and pacing in their cages. Animals kept indoors where high 'static electricity' levels exist, can exhibit signs of depression or become irritable due to excess of positive ions. For more information read "The Ion Effect", by Fred Soyka, Bantam Books, 1991.

For continuing information on alternative health care for pets, read Natural Pet Magazine PO Box 351, Trilby FL 33593-0351 (904)-583-2770.

For information on the holistic companion animal newsletter "Health Animals" by Dr. Robert Goldstein and Susan Goldstein call (203)-222-7173.

RESOURCE DIRECTORY

This directory provides information on non-toxic products which can help keep your pet healthy. Since many readers may not know where to find solutions mentioned in our chapters, we have described a variety of them and listed a resource to contact for further information.

SAFE CLEANERS/DEODORIZERS

SAFE ENVIRONMENTAL ODOR ELIMINATOR. A new product from Canada goes to the source of pet malodor (urine) and turns it to nitrogen, oxygen and water through a molecular change (ozone). Odor Out, available from Nature's Answers, is a liquid combination of oxidizer and yucca and is 2.5 times more powerful than chlorine. It kills bacteria and won't allow flea eggs to hatch or ringworm to spread. It gets rid of skunk odor. Other products provided include Psyllium Combination, herbal remedy for hairballs, Nature's Answers, 363 Carroll Close, Tarrytown, NY 10591 (800)-395-7134.

OLD FASHIONED UNSCENTED SAFE SOAPS. Coastline Products makes a variety of safe alternatives to laundry and dishwashing detergents, carpet shampoo and fabric stain removers. They are biodegradable and contain no formaldehyde, fragrance, phosphates, dye or harmful preservatives. Non-toxic if swallowed in diluted form. Coastline Products, P.O. Box 6397, Santa Ana, CA 92706, 800-554-4111.

A BOTANICAL SOLUTION TO ODOR POLLUTION. An all natural, safe, non-toxic, odorless air freshener and deodorizer, the Hygenaire uses vegetable and citrus extracts. It contains no cover-up scents, harmful fragrances or petrochemicals. Within the housing is a small fan which continually evaporates the solution into the air, reducing pet area and litter box odors. Lasting for six weeks or longer, the solution treats an area of 240 square feet. Allergy Alternatives, 440 Godfrey Dr., Windsor, CA 95492 (707)-838-1514.

NATURAL ZEOLITE MINERALS FOR ODOR. The minerals in ODORZOUT™ are mined in Arizona and have a honeycomb-like structure with pores which absorb and trap unpleasant odors. It is great in litter boxes, deters flea and tick infestation, may be sprinkled on dirt pet runs and in pet houses and is effective in removing skunk odors from your pet. It takes urine odors out of carpet, padding and flooring, and since it contains no chemicals or perfumes it is safe for people and pets. No Stink, 6020 W. Bell Rd. #E101, Glendale, AZ 85308, (800)-88STINK.

PET HEALTH

NATURAL PET FOOD. A healthy alternative to commercial pet foods, PetGuard contains no fillers, preservatives or animal byproducts. It comes in both canned and dry varieties for dogs and cats. PetGuard also produces Vegetarian canned food, Mr. Barky's vegetarian dog biscuits, natural food supplements and pet care products. PetGuard, Inc. PO box 728, Orange Park FL 32067-0728 (800)-874-3221.

OMEGA 3 WITHOUT FISH OIL. Essential fatty acids (Omega 3 & 6) are the building blocks of cell membranes and will help balance and normalize the body. Since they are processed out of most of our foods, we must use supplements. FORTIFIED FLAX provides these essential fatty acids with the oil in flax seed. It is nature's richest source of Omega-3 and this ground whole flax seed also contains all essential amino acids, high fiber, complex carbohydrates, vitamins and minerals. Omega-Life, Inc., PO Box 208, Brookfield, WI 53008-0208 (800)-EAT-FLAX (328-3529).

ALL NATURAL WHEAT KITTY LITTER. SWheat Scoop is a litter made from 100% whole wheat. Active enzymes in the wheat neutralize and destroy enzymes in cat urine which prevents the ammonia odor. It is dust free and contains no harmful silica or quartz dust, no absorbing clays, is flushable and biodegradable. Pet Care Systems, 717 N. Clinton, Grand Ledge, MI 48837 (800)-794-3287.

LIQUID MINERALS IN ELECTROLYTE SOLUTION. Trace minerals in crystalloid form are the key to continuing good health, shiny, healthy fur, good calcium absorption and a healthy disposition. PetLyte puts the life force back in food and water to fortify the body's defense against chemical additives. It is a blend of trace minerals in a base of distilled water. Naturopathic Research, P.O. Box 380175, Murdock, FL 33938-0175 (941)-426-5772.

THERAPEUTIC YUCCA PLANT. Used for centuries, the yucca plant is an excellent anti-inflammatory and proven to be a safe substitute for steroid-based medications. Yucca Intensive liquid is easy to feed to birds, rabbits, ferrets, cats, dogs, farm animals and horses. It can reduce pain and soft tissue inflammation, eliminates digestive problems, reduces allergic itch and can promote tissue healing and reduce scarring. Holistic Animal Care, 3150 N. Lodge Rd., Tucson, AZ 85715 (800)-497-5665.

GOURMET PET TREATS. Vermont Treats has a "cookie" factory on the island" in Bellows Falls, VT. There, they make all natural gourmet pet treats without chemicals, dyes or artificial preservatives. They currently offer tasty dog treats in humorous shapes such as peanut butter people, beef butterflies, liver unicorns, and also provide small and large bones. Treats for cats, horses and ferrets will be available soon. Vermont Treats, 1 Hapgood St., Bellows Falls, VT 05101 (802)-463-0711.

NATURE'S GREEN FOOD. Bright & Healthy Spirulina is a natural green food that builds strong immune systems and because of its chlorophyll content, can act as a natural antiseptic and rejuvenator. It contains concentrated amino acids, anti-oxidants and more, to satisfy your pet's requirement for live enzyme producing foods. Earthrise Animal Feeds, P.O. Box 818, Petaluma, CA 94953 (800)-995-0681.

ALL-NATURAL WILD BIRD FOOD. Created in cooperation with the National Wildlife Federation, Wings is the first super-premium, all-natural, fortified wild bird food. Wings is a high quality bird food, using only the best seeds with no artificial ingredients and no fillers like oats, rice, milo, or buckwheat. It has added vitamins, minerals, amino acids, enzymes and antioxidants. to help give birds a balanced meal. Sold in health food and eco stores and other specialty outlets. Natural World Interactions, Inc. PO Box 2250, Halesite, NY 11743. (800)-WINGS-67.

NATURE'S OWN FOLKLORIC REMEDY. Formulated for dogs and cats who are subject to the same bacteria, viruses or fungi that people are, Equilite and JBR Equine products contain a combination of herbs, vitamins and minerals which enhance overall health. GarliC contains Garlic, good against fleas and ticks; Astragalus, immune system strengthener; Schlsandra, good for coughs, wheezing, vitamin C and Zinc. Canine Balance assists in digestion, assimilation and detoxification and Canine Flex helps dogs with mobility problems (pain, stiffness). Equilite and JBR Equine Products, 20 Prospect Ave., Ardsley, NY 10502 (914)-693-2553.

ANTIOXIDANT AND IMMUNE SUPPORT. "Pet Formula Trace Minerals" is a veterinary designed, common sense approach to maximize your pets nutrition and enhance the immune system. Its trace minerals come from a multisource green food base, plant based digestive enzymes help to break down commercial pet foods, and the antioxidant complex slows the natural process of aging. It provides all the benefits of green foods and aids in flea control. Animal Food & Supply Co., PO Box 25092, Los Angeles, CA 90025 (800)-526-0065.

FORMULA FOR ALLERGIES AND SKIN. BIO-COAT is a concentrated biotin feed supplement for dogs and cats enriched with other vitamins and minerals in a base of primary dried yeast (not brewer's yeast). It is good for dry skin, dull thinning coats and scratching problems. BIO-COAT can be given to pets with allergies as a safe, effective and inexpensive nutritional adjunct to prednisone and cortisone and has no artificial colors, flavors or preservatives. Nickers International, Ltd., 12 Schubert St., Dept. B, Staten Island, NY 10305 (800)-642-5377.

PET VITAMINS. If your companion animal's health is compromised by food rich in fats, additives and preservatives, they definitely need clearing, detox and support. HomeoVetiX formulations have been developed by a pharmacist for natural pet care. They have been "human tested" since 1979 and intensify the innate healing energy of the animal. They are used for allergy and stress control as well as clearing, detoxification and nutritional support. HomeoVetiX, 3427 Exchange Ave., Naples, FL 33942 (800)-964-7177.

NATURAL HERBAL REMEDIES FOR DOGS. The best remedies often are nature's own which is the concept behind the first line of liquid herbal formulas for dogs. Tasha's Herbs for Dogs come in concentrated drops that are alcohol-free, palatable and include flower essences; Adult & Senior Support, The Traveler, Willow Bark Formula, Easy Does It, Skin & Hair Support. Coyote Springs Co., Box 1175, Jackson WY 83001 (800)-315-0142.

NUTRITIONAL SUPPLEMENTS FOR DOGS. Nutritional supplementation is needed to strengthen your dog's system. SOURCE PLUS! was designed to fortify your dog against increasing environmental stresses. Its all-natural ingredients include Dehydrated Seaweed Meals, Nutritional Yeast Cultures and Garlic Powder. When included in your dog's daily diet, you can expect improvements in allergies, skin and coat condition and overall health. SOURCE Inc., 101 Fowler Rd., North Branford, CT 06471 (800)-232-2365.

SUPER BLUE GREEN™ ALGAE. This green food supplies all the essential raw dietary nutrients that are lost in the processing of most animal foods. It is a wild food in a raw, synergistic, organic form providing vital dietary elements necessary for your pet's health. An economical way to get proper nutrition for your animal. Independent Distributors Sharon Trump and Dr. Philip Haselden, 14055 Bicky Rd., Orlando, FL 32824 (800)-808-7242.

NECESSARY WHOLE FOOD SUPPLEMENTS. Natural, whole food supplements are necessary for proper nutritional balance. Pines wheat grass powders or tablets are rich in vitamins, minerals, anti-oxidants and enzymes. This product nutritionally resembles a dark green leafy vegetable, but is much more concentrated. It should be a necessary part of your pet's daily diet. Pines International, P.O. Box 1107, Lawrence, KS 66044 (800)-697-4637.

GARLIC EXTRACT. The world's only truly odorless garlic that is aged to perfection is Kyolic®. Its unique aging process changes the harsh compounds and enhances the benefits found in raw garlic. Other valuable nutrients are found in Kyo-Green®, a blend of organically grown young barley and wheat grasses, Bulgarian chlorella and kelp. Wakunaga of America, Ltd., 23501 Madero, Mission Viejo, CA 91691 (800)-826-7888.

RAW ENZYMES/VITAMINS IN A GRAVY MIX. NUPRO users have had wonderful results with pets who have allergies, hot spots, arthritis, poor appetite, anemia, scratching and itching. This gravy forming mix (liver flavor) includes bee pollen, flaxseed, borage seed, lecithin, garlic, acidophilus, nutritional yeast, kelp. It has no ash, sugar, fillers, preservatives or by-products and is highly recommended by many healthy pets. Nutri Pet Research, Inc.,8 West Main St., Farmingdale, NJ 07727 (800)-360-3300.

ALLERGENIC SKIN CARE. Commercial pet shampoos can cause skin irritation and other problems. Espree has formulated effective grooming shampoos and conditioners with no detergents, insecticides or harmful drying or coat burning agents and is formulated to prevent the growth of potentially dangerous bacteria, fungi or other micro-organisms. Their products can help relieve flea bite dermatitis, itching, other skin problems and fur matting and tangling. Espree Animal Products, 6015 Commerce Dr., Suite 400, Irving, TX 75063 (800)-328-1317.

ENZYMATIC FOOD SUPPLEMENT. The absorption of essential nutrients and fatty acids from pet food are sometimes difficult, making it necessary to add enzymes to the pet's diet. Consisting of lipases, amylases, proteases and cellulases, Prozyme is beneficial to dogs, cats, birds, rabbits, horses, etc. It is all natural and scientifically tested to provide maximum absorption of nutrients needed by your animal. Prozyme Products, 6600 N. Lincoln Ave., Lincolnwood, IL 60645 (800)-522-5537.

FLEA & TICK POWDERS. Earth-safe, natural alternatives to harsh, potentially toxic chemicals and synthetic substitutes are the responsible way to protect your pet. Natural Animal, Inc. offers their pet care line which includes herbal shampoos, collars, natural pyrethrin-based flea and tick powders, vitamins, yeast and garlic supplements and biodegradable, flushable litter. Their home care line includes diatomaceous earth and natural pyrethrin-based insect powders. Natural Animal, Inc., 7000 US 1 North, St. Augustine, FL 32085 (800)-274-7387.

HOMEOPATHIC REMEDIES. 100% natural homeopathic pet treatments for anxiety, arthritis, cough, flea dermatitis, gastroenteritis, hot spot dermatitis, miliary eczema (male & female), sinusitis, skin and seborrhea, trauma, urinary infections and incontinence are available from HomeoPet. They all are F.D.A. registered, cruelty-free and contain no chemical residue. A safe alternative to injections and drugs, these remedies are formulated by veterinarians for cats and dogs (not for human consumption). HomeoPet, Westhampton Beach, NY 11978-0147 (800)-556-0738.

LIVING GREENS FOR INDOOR PETS. Most pets need the nutrition that green foods give them. Living foods have all their nutrients in tact. The Sproutsville Greens Kit for Pets, allows you to hydroponically grow clover for your bunnies, wheat or barley grass for your cats and dogs, etc. Let them munch or chop the greens up and add to their food. Sproutsville, PO Box 539, Otis, MA 01253 (413)-269-7307.

NATURAL MEDICINES WITHOUT SIDE EFFECTS. Dr. Goodpet offers natural homeopathic medicines that work without side effects, against fleas and insect bites, scratching, motion sickness, ear and eye problems. Also provides hypoallergenic vitamins and trace minerals specific for the very young, adults and seniors. Canine and feline digestive enzymes and hypoallergenic PURE shampoos are available as well. Dr. GOODPET LABORATORIES, Inc. Inglewood CA. (800)-222-9932.

PAIN RELIEF FOR HIP DYSPLASIA OR ARTHRITIS. Glyco-Flex (for dogs) and Nu-Cat (for cats) provides Perna Canaliculus, a safe and natural approach for relieving your pets discomfort due to hip dysplasia or arthritis. Your pet will gain a greater range of motion, increase in exercise tolerance and overall improvement in attitude. There are no side effects associated with these products. Sold through your Veterinarian. Vetri-Science Laboratories, 20 New England Dr., Essex Jct., VT 05453.

TRADITIONAL FLOWER REMEDIES. The calming essence and non-addictive effectiveness of flower remedies is well documented. These creams and liquids relieve emotional stress and imbalances, and can acts as excellent first aid products. Ellon's formulas have been used worldwide for over 60 years and were discovered by a British physician. Ellon USA, 644 Merrick Rd., LynBrook, NY 11563 (800)-4-BE-CALM (423-2256).

HELP FOR DRY SKIN AND SCRATCHING. If your pet is always scratching or itching you can give them a Halo Dream Coat food supplement. Not only will it relieve these problems, but it is guaranteed to help dry skin and dandruff as well. They also manufacture Naturally Free Pet Spray which is a non-chemical deterrent to fleas and other pests. Naturally Free by Bug-Off, Rt. 4, Box 4753, Shelburne, VT 05482 (802)-785-5601.

AIR TREATMENT

AIR PURIFIERS BY ALPINE. These units purify the air by emitting low levels of naturally occurring ozone along with negative ions. They literally zap pollution out of the air. Various sizes are available for confined spaces to whole house applications. They produce beneficial negative ions that can have a calming effect on pets. The Building Analyst, 283 East Canaan Rd., East Canaan, CT 06024 or a local Alpine representative.

AIR CLEANERS FROM AUSTIN. Whole house or whole kennel air cleaning occurs through the unit which is equipped with an 80 sq.ft. HEPA (high efficiency particulate arrestor) filter and 15 pounds of carbon filtration. This unit removes dust, most gases and bacteria down to .3 microns as the internal fan draws air through the machine. Aquarius Health, 7220 Porter Rd., Niagara Falls, NY 14304 (716) 298-4686.

OZONE PURIFIERS BY PANDA. Practical, small, lightweight ozone generators with negative ions that are useful in kennels and aviaries to prevent skin disorders and allergies. The Panda will eliminate pet odors, kill bacteria, neutralize cat dander and harmful air contamination caused by indoor pollution. No filters to change. Quantum Electronics, 110 Jefferson Blvd., Warwick, RI 02888 (800)-966-5575.

SILENT AIR TREATMENT. Developed in Japan to treat children with infantile asthma and people with allergies, the Clearveil electronic air cleaner operates silently, and works by releasing negative ions that attach themselves to airborne particles. It then attracts these contaminants to the unit with a positively charged collection sheet, which is easily changed each month. Excellent for odors, viruses, smoke, animal dander, mold fragments and bacteria. Clearveil Corp., 1660 17th St., Suite 200, Denver, CO 80202 (800)-531-6662.

WATER PURIFICATION

CARBON BASED COUNTERTOP WATER FILTER. Aqua Belle water purifier attaches to your faucet and provides protection from lead, chlorine, certain bacteria and sediment. A practical, inexpensive way to protect your pet from ill health due to water contamination. It's replaceable filters are good for two years. Aqua Belle Mfg., Co., P.O. Box 496, Highland Park, IL 60035, (708)-432-8979.

REVERSE-OSMOSIS (R/O) WATER SYSTEM. The Water Solution is a countertop R/O unit that provides fast delivery of pure water. It removes 98% of all contamination at the maximum rate of 100 gallons per day. Easily stored when not in use, this system is contained in a single housing and is adaptable to under the sink applications. The Building Analyst, 283 East Canaan Rd., East Canaan, CT 06024.

INDOOR ENVIRONMENTAL EDUCATION

BAU-BIOLOGIE & ECOLOGY COURSES. The objective of the International Institute for Bau-Biologie & Ecology is to make people aware of the environmental factors in living and work places that have adverse effects on their health and tells them what to do to overcome these problems. Throughout the US, they provide correspondence courses, classes, workshops and seminars leading to certification of Bau-Biologie Home Inspector, and also offer "healthy house" products. IBE, Box 387, Clearwater, FL 34615 (813)-461-4371

BUILDING AND DECORATING PRODUCTS

RADIANT HEAT PANELS. Enerjoy Solid state radiant electric heating panels are allergy-free and can act as supplemental heating to kennels and pet cages. Designed for whole house usage, these units operate at 50% of the cost of normal electric heat. They are easy to install by an electrician and operate efficiently in well insulated homes. SSHC, Inc. PO Box 769, Old Saybrook CT 06475 (203)-388-3848.

FULL SPECTRUM LIGHTING. This type of lighting is the closest to natural sunlight. It provides pets with a natural bright light and heat source that closely mimics the spectrum of natural sunlight. The extra long life Lumichrome bulb emits beneficial Ultraviolet rays. This type of lighting is essential to preventing depression in kennels and homes during the winter. M. Pencar Associates, 137-75 Geranium Ave., Flushing, NY 11355 (800)-788-5781.

DO-IT-YOURSELF TESTING KITS FOR LEAD. Test your painted surfaces, dishes, toys, etc. for lead paint with LeadCheck Swabs, and test your water for lead down to 15 ppb (EPA reg.), with LeadCheck Aqua. These self-test kits give you results immediately as there is nothing to mail away. An 800 help line can advise you of stores nearby that carry these test kits and give you advice on your test results. HybriVet Systems, Inc. PO Box 1210, Framingham, MA 01701 (800)-262-5323.

NON-ELECTRIC ROOM HUMIDIFIER. All animals stay healthier with proper indoor humidity. This unit affixes to your electric or hot water baseboard heating unit and passively evaporates moisture. It needs no electricity, no demineralization cartridges, and can use regular tap water. As a no maintenance appliance, it is truly energy efficient. VP Enterprise, 98 Elmira Ave., Torrington, CT 06790 (203)-482-2441.

NON-TOXIC PAINTS/SEALERS. It is necessary to Protect yourself and your pets from harmful chemical fumes when you paint or refinish wood. Non-toxic Crystal Aire Sealers and Crystal Shield Paints are water soluable and block out formaldehyde, molds and other toxic emmissions. Allergy Alternatives, 440 Godfrey Dr., Windsor, CA 95492 (800)-838-1514.

HOME TESTING KITS. To protect your animals from harmful indoor pollutants you must first verify if they are present in your home. Tests for water, radon, lead and carbon monoxide available. Enzone Inc., 4800 SW 51st St., Bldg #100, Davie FL 33314 (800)-448-0535.

MISCELLANEOUS

NATURAL WORMER. There is a safe product that helps your pet resume their normal activities by ridding their body of digestive worms. Solid Gold Homeopet Wormer consists of natural herbs which remove the physical environment that the worm needs to survive. It contains no chemicals or poisons therefore is safe for your pet. Also available are Solid Gold natural dog and cat food and nutritional supplements. Dubl-K-Pet, PO Box 1871, Mishawaka, IN 46546. (800)-382-5573.

HOME STUDY REMEDIES. For more information on homeopathic and natural remedies this company has a myriad of videos, books and home study courses on the following subjects: Herbs, Flower remedies, Gem essence, Acupressure, Chiropractic, Massage, Sports therapies, working dogs and other alternative therapies. Advanced Animal Concepts for Alternative Solutions, 2152 Hazlitt Dr., Houston, TX 77032 (800)-228-8768.

BIBLIOGRAPHY

"**A Dish Owner's Guide to Potential Lead Hazards**," free from the Environmental Defense Fund, 5655 College Ave.,Oakland, Calif. 94618

"**A Guide to Indoor Air Quality**", U.S. Environmental Protection Agency, US Consumer Product Safety Commission, 1988

"**A Homebuyer's Guide To Environmental Hazards**", US Environmental Protection Agency, et al.

Amdt, Linda, "**The Reintroduction of Whole Living Foods**", Natural Pet Magazine, Mar/Apr. 1995

Ackerman, Lowell, DVM, "**Enzyme Therapy in Veterinary Practice**", Advances in Nutrition, Vo. 1, No. 3, 1993

Anderson, Nina & Benoist, Albert: **Your Health and Your House**; Keats Publishing, 1995

Anonymous: **N,N-diethyl-m-toluamide (DEET)**; Pesticide registration standard, US EPA, Office of Pesticide and Toxic Substances, Wash. DC 1980

Aontine, W.J., and Uno, T.: **Acute aspirin toxicity in a cat**; Vet. Med. Sm. Anim. Clin., 64:680, 1969

Atkins, Clarke E., DVM, Johnson, Roger K.,DVM, "**Clinical Toxicities of Cats**", Veterinary Clinics of North America, Vol. 5, No. 4

Beasley, Val R., D.V.M., PhD, Guest Editor, The Veterinary Clinics of North America, Small Animal Practice, Vo. 20/ No. 2, March 1990: **Toxicology of Selected Pesticides, Drugs, and Chemicals**; W.B. Saunders Co.

Bodanis,David: **The Secret House**; Simon & Schuster, Washington and Beyond, 1986.

"**Can Your House Make You Sick**", Popular Science, July 1992

"**Carbon Monoxide, a Silent Hazard**", Home Ecology, Home Magazine, Oct. 1993.

"**Carbon Monoxide Poisoning**", Medical Essay, Mayo Clinic Health Letter, February 1984

"Carboxyhemoglobin Levels in Patients with Flu-Like Symptoms", Annals of Emergency, Medicine, July 1987

Casaida JE, Gammon DW, Glickman AH: Mechanisms of selective action of pyrethroid insecticides; Annu Rev Pharmacol Toxicol 23:413-438, 1983

Case, Penny, **"Flower Power"**, Natural Pet Magazine, Nov/Dec. 1994

Claiborne Ray, C., **"Teflon and Parrots,"** Science Times, The New York Times, Feb. 1995

Clarke, E.G.C.: **Lead poisoning in small animals**; J. Sm. Anim. Pract., 14:183, 1973

Coppock RW, Mostrom MS, Lillie LE: **The toxicology of detergents, bleaches, antiseptics and disinfectants in small animals**; Vet Hum Toxicol 30:463-473, 1988

"Contaminant Alert", Executive Report, Water Technology, Jan. 1993

Cremer JE: **The influence in mammals of the pyrethroid insecticides**; Dev Toxicol Environ Sci ll:61-72, 1983

Dadd, Debra Lynn, **"Put Your Foot Down to Toxic Carpets"**, Earth Star, Feb./Mar. 1993

"EPA Says 819 Public Water Systems Pose Lead Risk", Water Technology magazine, July 1993.

Ertel, Grace, **"The Booming Bug eat Bug Industry,"** In Business magazine, Jan/Feb. 1995

"Getting the Lead Out of Your Water", Better Homes and Gardens, May 1992

Goodman, Jerry, **"The Alternatives to Modern Pest Control"**, Healthy & Natural Journal, Vol 2, No.1

Gosselin RE, Smith RP, Hodge HC: **Clinical Toxicology of Commercial Products**, ed 5. Baltimore, Williams & Wilkins, 1984,

Greeley, Alexandra, **"Getting the Lead Out of Just About Everything"**, FDA Consumer, July/August 1991

Greer, J.M.: Plant poisoning in cats;. Mod. Vet. Pract., 42:62, 1961

"Heat Recovery Ventilation for Housing", U.S. Dept. Energy, Appropriate Technology Program, 1984

Hellmich, Nanci, "Experts urge lead tests for household taps", USA Today, Jan. 19, 1993

Hoffman, Ronald L., M.D., "Chronic Fatigue Syndrome Update", New Life Magazine, Mar/April 1993

"Household cleaners, pest control", Housatonic Current, Spring 1994

"Is your water safe?", US News and World Report, Jul 29, 1991

Krenzelok EP: "Liquid automatic diswashing detergents: A profile of toxicity" Ann Emerg Med 18:60-63. 1989

Larson, E.J. " Toxicity of low doses of aspirin in the cat." J.A.V.M.A., 143;837, 1963

"Lead-Based paint Disclosures Are Now Mandatory", Good Cents Magazine, Jan/Feb

Lee JF, Simonowitz D, Block GE, "Corrosive injury of the stomach and esophagus by nonphosphate detergents". Am J Surg 123:652-656, 1972

Martlew, Gillian, N.D. "Electrolytes, The Spark of Life", Nature's Publishing, 1994

Martlew, Gillian, N.D., "Is Your Pet Missing Out?", Naturopathic Research, 1994

Meyerowitz, Steve, "Water, Pollution. Purification", Sprout House, 1990

Moffatt,Sebstian, "Backdrafting Woes", Progressive Builder Dec. 1986

"Moisture and Home Energy Conservation", Energy Administration Clearinghouse, Michigan Dept. Commerce

Newman, Lisa, "Great Clumping Cat Litter..Is That Why Kitty Is So Sick?", Natural Pet Magazine, Mar/Apr. 1995

"News from CPSC", US Consumer Product Safety Commission, May 31, 1990

Oehme, Frederick W., D.V.M., Ph.D., Guest Editor; The Veterinary Clinics of North America; Vol 5/ #4, Nov. 1075, **"Symposium on Clinical Toxicology for the Small Animal Practitioner"**, W.B. Saunders Co.

O'Brien, Robert, **"Magic Ions in the Air"**, Alpine Air, 1991

Pedersen, Mike, **"POE Systems Reduce VOC Risks"**, Water Technology, Aug. 1994

Pencar, Mark, **"Lighten Up"**, Natural Pet Magazine, Jul/Aug 1994

"Pet Care Tips", Ralston Purina Co., 1994

Petrak, M.L.: **Diseases of Cage and Aviary Birds**; Philadelphia, Lea & Febiger, 1969

Pinckney,Edward, M.D.,**"Carbon Monoxide Poisoning in the Home"**, Vector Consumer Newsletter, Nov. 8, 1988

Priester, W.A., and Hayes, H.M.: **Lead poisoning in cattle, horses, cats and dogs as reported by 11 colleges of veterinary medicine in the US and Canada**; from July, 1968 through June, 1972. Am. J. Vet. Res., 35:567, 1974

Ramsey, F.K., et al,: **Diagnostic aspects of diseases produced by toxicants in small animals**; Anim. Hosp., 3:221, 1967

Radeleff, R.D.: **Veterinary Toxicology**; Philadelphia, Lea & Febiger, 1964

Rees, Ann, **"Chlorinated Water Linked to Cancer, study shows"**, The Province, July 2, 1992

"Renovating Your Home Without Lead Poisoning Your Children", Conservation Law Foundation, Dept. L, 3 Joy St., Boston, Mass. 02108.

"Report concludes fluoridated water is safe", Industry Watch, Water Technology magazine, Oct, 1993

Reyes, Consuelo, **"In our own backyards!"**, Cancer Forum, Vol.13, No. 5/6

Riotte, Louise: **Carrots Love Tomatoes**; Garden Way Publishing, 1981

Robb, Maribeth Murphy, **"The True Cost of Hard Water"**, Kitchens and Bath magazine, July 1991.

Robbins PJ, Cherniack MG: **Review of the biodistribution and toxicity of the insect repellent N,N-diethyl-m-toluamide (DEET)**; J Toxicol Environ Health 18:503-525-1986

Rousseaux CG, Smith RA, Nicholson S: **Acute Pine Sol toxicity in a domestic cat**; Vet Hum Toxicol 28:3160317, 1986

"Safer Cleaning Products", Washington Toxics Coalition, Seattle, Wa.

Scott, H.M.: **Lead poisoning in small animals**; Vet. Rec., 75:830, 1963

Smith, Charlene, **"Green Foods"**, Natural Pet Magazine, May/June 1994

Smith, Charlene, **"How to treat Common Conditions with Herbs"**, Natural Pet Magazine, May/June 1994.

Soyka, Fred, **" The Ion Effect"**, Bantam, 1991

Sprung, C. and Kaskin, S.T.; **Our panel reports**; Mod. Vet. Pract., 51:42, 1970

"Straight Answers to Burning Questions", Wood Heating Alliance, 1101 Connecticut Ave NW, Suite 700, Washington, DC 20036

Taylor, Alfred, **"Fluoride and Cancer"**, Saturday Review, Oct. 2, 1965

Temple AF: **Bleach, soaps and detergents**; In Haddad LM, Winchester JF (eds): Clinical Management of Poison and Drug Overdose. Philadelphia, WB Saunders, 1983

"Treating EPA Regulated Water Contaminants", Water Technology magazine, Directory Issue, 1995

Wasserman, B.: **Sheep laurel poisoning in the cat - A case report**;, J.A.V.M.A. 135:569, 1959

Weissman, Art & Lisa R. Kruse, **"Lead threat may hit 1 in 6"**, Asbury Park Press Statehouse Bureau, N.J., Aug. 5, 1993

"What everyone should know about Lead Poisoning", State of Connecticut Dept. Health Svc.

"What is Antifreeze?", California Integrated Waste Management Board, Sacramento, CA

Wilkinson, G.T.,: **A review of drug toxicity in the cat**; J.SM. Anim. Pract., 9:21, 1968

"Your Drinking Water - How Good is it?", National Testing Laboratories, Cleveland Ohio.

References to herbal cures:
"Understanding and Choosing Herbal Products", Charlene Smith, Natural Pet Magazine, May/June 1994.
Potter's New Cyclopaedia of Botanical Drugs and Preparations by R.C. Wren
The Complete Herbal Handbook for Farm & Stable by Juliette de Bairacli Levy
Todays Herbal Health by Louise Tenney
Prescription for Nutritional Healing by James F. Balch, MD
The Scientific Validation of Herbal Medicine by Daniel B. Mowrey, Ph.s.
The Little Herb Encyclopedia, by J. Ritchason
Your Cat Naturally, Grace Mchattie, Carroll & Graf Publishers, NY

INDEX

exercise (7, 29, 81, 84, 105)
eyelid blinking (6)
Fennel (91)
fertilizers (4, 48, 58)
fireplaces (27, 28, 33)
flea control (6, 11, 102)
fluoride (7, 54, 58, 62-64, 67, 114)
foggers (2, 11, 12)
formaldehyde (5, 7, 20, 70, 72, 74, 75, 99, 109)
fuel oil (22)
full spectrum lights (78)
fumigation (11)
G-H
garden (5, 6, 8, 113)
garlic (12, 66, 83, 88, 90, 91, 102-105)
gastroenteritis (3, 7, 22, 49, 50, 105)
growling (37)
hair loss (17, 20, 94)
head tremors (3, 6)
heart disease (87)
heat recovery ventilators (32)
heavy metals (58, 83)
HEPA (79, 96, 106)
herbs (7, 11, 87, 88, 90, 91, 102, 103, 114)
"hormonal" pollutants (16)
humidity (75, 109)
hyperexcitability (7)
hypersalivation (7)
hyperthermia (17)
hysteria (37, 40)
I-L
infertility (2, 3)
IPM (8)
irritability (3-5, 26, 29, 71, 78)
laundry products (18, 19)
lead (5-7, 22, 35-46, 54, 58, 60-62, 67, 76, 82, 107-114)
lead in water (6, 41)
lead paint (5, 6, 36, 38-41, 43-46, 60, 76, 108)
lead pipes (38, 41, 42, 44, 61)
Lemon grass (8, 12, 23)
lemon juice (23)
lily (7, 51)
lindane (5)
listlessness (3, 6)
lung (91, 104)
M-N

malignant lymphoma (4)
methylene chloride (76)
minerals (7, 8, 55, 66, 81, 85, 86, 94, 100-103, 105)
mold (4, 5, 78, 79, 107)
mosquitos (8)
moth balls (22)
NAPCC (52)
nausea (3, 7, 9, 22, 26, 29, 30, 71, 74)
negative ions (79, 96, 97, 106, 107)
nervousness (3, 9, 71, 74)
nitrates (54, 58, 64)
nutritional yeast (11, 12, 83, 103, 104)
O-P
outgassing (69, 70, 74)
ozone (60, 76, 79, 96, 99, 106, 107)
paint (4-7, 15, 23, 27, 36, 38-41, 43-46, 60, 69, 75, 76, 96, 108, 109, 112)
panting (17, 20)
paralysis (3, 7, 22, 91)
parsley (83, 88, 90)
pennyroyal (11, 12)
pesticides (1-8, 10, 11, 16, 48, 54, 57-59, 65, 67, 78, 83, 110)
philodendron (50, 51)
Pine oil (20)
poisonous meals (5)
proteins (66, 86, 87)
pyrethrins (7)
Q-R
radon (109)
rat poison (6, 9, 62)
regurgitation (3, 7)
respiratory (3-7, 10, 18, 22, 29, 76, 78, 83, 91, 95)
restlessness (9, 17, 22, 37, 40, 56, 60)
ruffled feathers (3, 7)
S
sabadilla (7)
seagulls (2)
seizures (3, 5, 7, 10, 17, 20)
shock (17, 20)
skin conditions (92, 94)
Slippery elm (91)
soap (6, 19, 22, 45)
spiders (73)
stiffness (3, 6, 86, 102)
strychnine poisoning (6)
sunlight (7, 77, 108)
T-Z